The Challenge of Epilepsy

Take Control of Your Seizures—and Your Life—through Complementary and Alternative Solutions

by Sally Fletcher, MA

Aura Publishing Company

P.O. Box 6776, San Rafael, CA 94903-6776

www.epilepsyhealth.com

Notice and Disclaimer

This book is based on personal experience and observations. It is meant to be educational in nature and is not designed to instruct anyone in complete self-treatment, let alone diagnosis. Keep in mind that epilepsy is highly individualistic.

To learn about the latest advances in medication or surgery for epilepsy, seek out the best medical assistance you can find from a neurologist.

Former editions 1985 and 1986

Published by Aura Publishing Company, P.O. Box 6776, San Rafael, CA 94903-6776

Printed in the United States of America

Library of Congress Control Number: 2003095885

ISBN 0-9615513-6-4

Publisher's Cataloging-in-Pubication data

Fletcher, Sally

The Challenge of epilepsy / Take control of your seizures and your life through complementary and alternative solutions / Sally Fletcher. – 3rd ed.

123p. ill. 15 cm. X 23 cm.

Rev. ed. of : The Challenge of epilepsy / Sally Fletcher. 2nd ed.

Includes bibliographical references and index.

ISBN 0-9615513-6-4

1.Epilepsy. 2. Epilepsy—Social aspects. 3. Epilepsy—Patients. 4. Epilepsy—Family relationships. 5. Epilepsy—Popular works. 6. Epilepsy—Treatment.

RC372.2 F53 2003

616.853-dc21   2003095885

This book is for:

The millions of people who have seizures and who are searching for new and better ways to handle the problem;

The millions of people who have a loved one with epilepsy and want to know more about the disorder; and for

The neurologists, biofeedback and neurofeedback practitioners, receptionists, psychologists, social workers, counselors, teachers and nurses who show concern for their patients, clients or students by continuous learning.

Dedication

To my children, Kim and Michael Ray.

Together we grew to understand the meaning of words such as: disabled, poverty, prejudice, fear, anger, embarrassment, frustration, hope, perseverance, courage, compassion and love.

Acknowledgments

I wish to express special thanks to the following people, whose guidance, support and inspiration made this book possible:

Ron Petersen, Robert Shellenberger, Ph.D., and John Turner, Ph.D., for their unselfish help and guidance as I experimented with and practiced biofeedback training at the Aims Biofeedback Institute in Greeley, Colorado.

Judith Green, Ph.D., Sidney Kurn, M.D., and Merritt Lewis, who gave me unending inspiration and encouragement for the first writing of this book.

Roxanne Preble, M.A., neurofeedback practitioner, and Susan Rosen, for sharing their knowledge and expertise regarding neurofeedback.

Kim Spencer for her meticulous proofreading, support and suggestions (both humorous and serious).

Richard Bagel of Richard Bagel Design Studios, for cover and interior design and layout.

Michael Bremer of UnTechnical Press, for editing and publishing consulting.

Table of Contents

Chapter 1

How I Learned About Epilepsy

Many years of my life were spent searching for a simple, miraculous, instantaneous cure for my epilepsy.

I eventually became free of seizures, but it wasn't instantaneous. I now believe that many people's seizures can be reduced, or even eliminated, by gradual life-style changes, including proper nutrition and stress management, along with neurofeedback (EEG biofeedback) training and other techniques. It doesn't usually happen overnight; change can be complex and no one can do it for you. Developing new habits for your mind and body takes persistence, but the rewards affect your entire life.

The methods in this book are considered *alternative* or *complementary* to traditional healing (medicine and/or surgery). For information and questions related to medication and/or surgery, check with your physician. These alternative methods are: stress management, nutrition, exercise, yoga, self-esteem building, music, meditation, visualization, psychophysiology (biofeedback), and most importantly, accepting and learning to use the power of the mind. They are applicable to any disorder, "challenge" or disease. There are many other alternative therapies which you may want to look into as well. The word disease (dis-ease) means the absence of ease, comfort or health. We are souls living in our bodies, and the better we take care of ourselves, the more enjoyment we will experience in our lives.

This knowledge and wisdom wasn't something I was told by a physician, heard in a lecture hall, read in a book, or envisioned. My years of searching, much of it by trial and error, were not simply because of my humanitarian urge to wipe out epilepsy for the 2 – 6% of our population who live with seizures.[1] (Not that I wouldn't like that!) My motivation was the fact that I was experiencing l0 to l5 seizures per month which were uncontrolled by medication. I am now free of seizures, and I want to share what I have learned with you.

After my first seizure, at the age of 26, I made an appointment with a physician. Many questions were asked as the physician searched for, first of all, a diagnosis, then the cause of my disorder. The question, "Have you ever suffered a concussion or blow to the head?" provided a very important clue in the search.

I replied, "Yes, I suffered a concussion as the result of a fall while ice skating when I was 16." The physician suggested that I have an electroencephalogram (EEG) to gather data about my brain wave patterns, as well as a CAT Scan (computerized axial tomography) to see if there were any structural abnormalities in the brain. The CAT Scan did not reveal any abnormalities. The EEG test, which lasted three hours, showed a sharp spike and wave pattern in the left temporal lobe, which is common for many people with complex partial seizures. The physician's conclusion, after many hours of consultation, examination and probing, was that the sharp spikes in the brain wave pattern were from scar tissue, the scar tissue probably the result of the concussion 10 years earlier. Though my doctor tried prescription after prescription, no medication worked to completely control the seizures without horrible side effects.

I didn't believe the diagnosis—epilepsy—for several months. I referred to my seizures as "blackout spells" and made sure that everyone else use the term "spell" rather than "seizure." Many months of "spells" later, however, I finally had to face it; I had epilepsy.

The next 10 years were like a scene out of a horror movie. Although I am an accomplished musician and teacher and have scored above the 98th percentile on IQ tests, people treated me as if I were incompetent.

I wouldn't admit that it was unsafe to drive until I caused two accidents within five days, totaling six cars (but fortunately harming no one). The same police officer came to the scene both times. When he recognized me the second time, he asked for my driver's license and didn't give it back.

Then I lost my job. The worst day of my life was when I had to register for Supplemental Security Income (SSI), admitting that I could no longer earn a living or support my two children. My children and I lived in poverty. I was taking a lot of medication. I hardly knew what I was doing, and I was still having seizures.

I finally decided to fight back. I realized that rather than living, I was only non-dying. I could not undo the skating accident, and since medication didn't work for me, I had to find other options.

For years, I devoted myself to learning everything I could about epilepsy. Much time was spent examining my life—from the time when I first started having seizures to the time when I had the last one. I recorded on the calendar with a red X each time I had a seizure. I kept a journal, writing down how I was feeling, what I had been doing, eating and thinking, and when a seizure would occur. After a few years of collecting information I could see a pattern which showed when and why seizures occurred for me.

Stress (my reaction to stressors) was the number one cause. Pressure for time, disagreements, arguments, an excess of worry, indecision, fear and excitement were closely linked to seizures. The seizure often occurred a day or two after the stress. Skipping meals and consuming too much sugar, caffeine or alcohol would often trigger a seizure. Or a seizure would occur after a night of insufficient sleep. I had more seizures the week before and during menstruation than the rest of the month.

I also talked and corresponded with hundreds of people with epilepsy. From this I learned about habits, thoughts, feelings and lifestyles, and received many helpful suggestions from others who have seizures.

I read every book, article and pamphlet about epilepsy that I could find. I discovered that the literature on epilepsy is limited. Much of the information describes the various types of seizures, the medications available, brain surgery, and what to do when you or someone else has a seizure. This information was helpful, but I wanted more. I was searching for information on how to overcome epilepsy—how to reduce or eliminate seizures using unconventional (alternative or complementary) methods.

I learned to control my seizures gradually, experimenting with many different methods. When one method didn't seem to help, I dropped it, then tried another—then another—then another. I believe it was a combination of methods that helped me to overcome my seizures. These methods were: neurofeedback (EEG biofeedback), positive thinking, developing more self esteem, yoga (both postures and meditation), correct nutrition, stress management, spirituality, music and regular exercise.

I still don't know which, if any, of these methods is most important. Each is an aid to the others, and they all work together. Since we human beings are unique, different methods and different combinations work for different people.

Having a seizure is very embarrassing, both to the person having it and to those who witness it. One person who has frequent seizures described this feeling of embarrassment very well. She says, "Have you ever slipped on ice and fallen on the street? Remember how you picked yourself up and looked around to see if anyone saw you? It wasn't your fault any more than having seizures is my fault, but why did you check to see if anyone saw you if the embarrassment of being seen didn't exist? Believe me, having a seizure is much more embarrassing than just slipping on ice!"

One of my most severe seizures occurred while I was teaching a group of yoga students a rapid deep-breathing exercise. (I now realize that hyper-ventilation can trigger seizures.) I came out of the seizure with blood running down my chin, crying, not knowing where I was or what had happened. The students were shocked and frightened, and I was only half-conscious, so some of them took me home. It took all of my courage to go back and face those students at the next class!

Sometimes during a complex partial (psychomotor) seizure I would pace back and forth, counting my steps aloud, or dance around singing a repetitive phrase. (Now that I'm a professional musician full time, I wonder if I should have recorded some of the singing; maybe they would be hit songs! Who knows?!) Seriously, this was very embarrassing, both to those around me and to myself, especially later when witnesses would tell me about these experiences, of which I was unaware.

The following scene is a personal experience. A young man who works at a laundromat near a downtown street corner is standing outside taking a break. Suddenly a woman walking toward him stops, stiffens, lets out a scream. She rolls her eyes, peels off her blouse, then starts singing, skipping and dancing. She twirls the blouse around as her right arm jerks and makes circles. The young man is terrified and fascinated.

"Is she on drugs? Is she psychotic? Is she dangerous? What shall I do?" As she comes out of the seizure he asks her a few questions and finally she answers. She mumbles something about epilepsy after he tells her what happened. She puts on her blouse and walks on home, her thinking fuzzy. She crawls into bed and falls asleep. Embarrassing episodes such as these served as an incentive to find a way to overcome seizures.

Being without a driver's license also gave me the desire to find a way to become free of seizures. Since there was no bus system in the city where I lived, I either walked or relied on others for transportation. Thinking of people to call, making phone calls, and arranging and waiting for rides sometimes took more time than the actual trip. I gained a lot of wisdom during those years of being dependent on others for rides, being restricted from most employment opportunities, and sometimes needing to rely on total strangers for help during a seizure.

I have always valued freedom, independence and self-sufficiency. I learned that living goes much more smoothly when I am willing to give and accept help from others when it is needed. For me this meant I had to swallow my pride and ask for rides—thousands of times. I learned the meaning of interdependence. I am very grateful for all the help I received. I want to repay some of this consideration by sharing what I have learned with as many people as possible.

The loss of memory which I experienced was another factor in making me determined to find a way to overcome epilepsy. Loss of memory can sometimes be a side effect of medication, and it can also be a result of the epilepsy itself. I noticed loss of memory especially after a seizure, then it would gradually improve until it was back to normal. This gradual change would sometimes take many days. When I had several seizures in one day or within a few days, I would remember very little of what had happened during that time. Even when I was free of seizures for two or three weeks, I would have lapses of memory. Sometimes I could recall the forgotten incident, name, etc., when someone described it. At other times it was completely gone from my memory. Some of the medication would also affect my memory and make my thinking disorganized and slow.

I spent several years of my life coping with the embarrassment from having seizures, the dependence and limitations of being without a driver's license, and from loss of memory. All of this made me determined not only to find a way to become seizure-free, but to become seizure-free *with the use of little or no medication*. I have now been free of seizures with no medication for over 15 years.

Ultimately, I learned that I was the one who needed to do the work in overcoming my problems. Physicians have studied many years so they can give suggestions and prescriptions to try to control the symptoms.

Since I was aware that medication was sometimes helpful, I used these suggestions from the physician when they seemed to fit my needs. If not, I found it wise to talk with the physician, sharing my thoughts and feelings, asking questions, trying to find the best solution for me to become healthier.

The neurologist whom I was seeing didn't know what I was doing 24 hours a day, didn't know what I had been eating, when and how often I felt stress, anger, boredom, frustration, or how I would feel on the days when I had seizures. So I learned that communication with the neurologist was very important. The neurologist could get a general idea of my well being by an examination and consultation; still, the person responsible for my well-being was (and still is) myself. Epilepsy is my challenge.

If you develop more self-esteem and understanding of epilepsy from reading this book, I will feel that my efforts have been worthwhile. Idealistically, I would like to see every person who has epilepsy become seizure-free and off medication. Realistically, I would like to see every person attain more self-awareness and self-esteem, adopting a healthy life-style which would make living (whether with or without epilepsy) a better experience.

----

[1] *The Epilepsy Fact Book,* Harry Sands and Frances C. Minters, (NY: Scribner, 1979) pp. 18-19.

Chapter 2

Some Myths And Facts About Epilepsy

From Myth to Modern Times

There are many ancient myths about epilepsy, and some of those superstitions still remain. Throughout history, individuals have been afflicted with seizures—mysterious fits during which they would sometimes fall to the ground and twitch convulsively, or wander about aimlessly, repeating some meaningless motor movement. People who most of the time were perfectly normal, happy and intelligent would suddenly appear to have become bewitched, possessed or seized by demons when a seizure overtook them. Why else would they foam at the mouth, jerk uncontrollably and be unaware of what had happened until someone later told them about the event.

As people ceased to believe in witchcraft, some other myths grew up to explain the phenomenon of epilepsy. Some thought it was caused by sins of the parents or by masturbation. Some said it led to insanity or feeble-mindedness. Laws were passed in many states forbidding people with epilepsy to marry or have children.

Many of the family members of people with epilepsy still refuse to talk about the disorder with friends and neighbors. Those who have seizures frequently try to hide this from others, feeling shame, as though there were some disgrace attached to epilepsy.

Today, even though there is still much to be learned about epilepsy, there is much information to show the truth. Many individuals are unaware of the facts.

Each year 100,000 new cases of epilepsy are reported in the United States. More than 2,000,000 Americans are believed to have epilepsy.[1] Epilepsy affects more people than cerebral palsy, cancer, tuberculosis, muscular dystrophy and multiple sclerosis combined.[2]

Brain and Body

Often, even those with epilepsy are unaware of just how the disorder wreaks its havoc on the body. Here's a brief explanation and additional background for those who want or need to understand more:

The central nervous system (often referred to as the CNS) consists of the brain and spinal cord. The spinal cord is a column of nerve tissue which joins with the lower part of the brain. The cord is enclosed by a bony structure called the spinal column. Nerves enter or leave the spinal cord through openings between the vertebra that compose the spinal column. These nerve fibers transmit impulses between the brain and other regions of the body. Motor impulses are directed from the brain to spinal nerves, then to the proper tissues for action. The body depends on the spinal cord for communication from the brain.

The brain is divided into three basic parts: the cerebrum, the cerebellum, and the brain stem. The cerebrum, the major portion of the brain, is the center of thinking and consciously-controlled activities. The motor area is the origin of purposeful actions. The cerebrum is divided into two physically separate halves, called "hemispheres." Each hemisphere relates to the opposite half of the body. For example, the sensation and movement of the right hand are accomplished by certain parts of the left hemisphere of the brain. Each hemisphere is subdivided into four major areas, called "lobes." Each lobe is responsible for vital functions. The outer half-inch of the brain is known as the cerebral cortex.

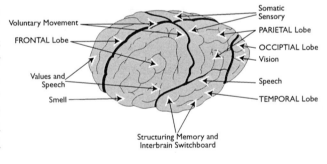

Beneath the cerebrum is the cerebellum, which monitors and coordinates body movements.

Next to the cerebellum is the brain stem, which connects with the spinal cord below and the cerebrum above. The brain stem carries nerve impulses from the cerebrum to the spinal cord and helps body processes such as breathing, circulation and digestion.

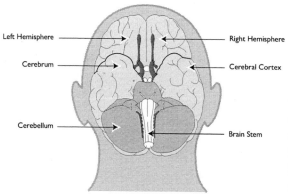

The cells that make up the brain are known as "neurons," or nerve cells. They are part of the tissue forming the central nervous system. There are millions of neurons in the brain and spinal cord.

Each neuron has three parts: the cell body, the dendrites, and the axon. Dendrites are fibers with many branches. They serve as receivers, picking up electrical impulses that are transmitted from other cells. Axons, which form the "tail" of the nerve, serve as the transmitters. They pass on information, in the form of electrical impulses to other cells. The electrochemical reactions by which the brain operates take place within the cell body itself.

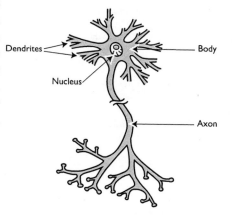

Neurons are information processors as well as transmitters and receivers. One of their functions is to block useless information. Sometimes a few neurons do not function correctly, setting up a chain reaction of indiscriminate firing. This can be the cause of a seizure.

Seizure Thresholds

Anyone who has some defect within the brain will be more vulnerable to epileptic seizures during times of tension or stress. This is called having a low seizure threshold, which is a term used to describe a level of tension or stress above which a certain person will have a seizure.

The potential to have a seizure exists in all of us; anyone can develop epilepsy, but the person who has a high seizure threshold will likely go through life without ever experiencing a convulsion.

Some things that can lower the threshold level or act as seizure precipitants are:

- Emotional stress, such as: divorce, death of someone close, anxiety, embarrassment or fear, feeling bad about oneself (80 – 90% of seizures are caused by stress.)

- Excitement

- Boredom, lack of activity or interest

- Extreme fatigue

- Lack of adequate, regular sleep

- Poor nutrition (eating junk food or skipping meals)

- Hypoglycemia (low blood sugar)

- Consumption of alcohol

- Heat and/or humidity

- Consumption of large amounts of food or drink at one time

- Allergies

- Menstrual cycle

- Bladder too full (putting off urination)

- Constipation

- Fever, colds, infections

- Drug abuse, especially with "uppers" such as PCP (phencyclidine hydrochloride) and amphetamines

- Drug withdrawal from "downers," barbiturates, Valium or alcohol

- Missed medication dosages

- Drug toxicity (too much medication)

- Sensory stimulation such as: sudden loud noise or sudden flashing lights

- Many more things too numerous to mention, and others that are still unknown

Causes

The causes of epilepsy vary, and for many people the cause is unknown. In epilepsy some brain cells discharge when they aren't supposed to, but the important question is why this happens. Some of the things which cause an individual to have a low seizure threshold (be more likely to have seizures than the average person) are: acquired, congenital and hereditary diseases; birth or pre-birth trauma (injuries); abnormal metabolism; chemical imbalance; allergies, and occasionally degenerative diseases affecting the brain.

Other causes can include poisoning (of which lead is the most common); brain tumors (less than 10 – 15%); CNS (central nervous system) infections, such as meningitis and encephalitis; scar formation in the brain from head injury or operation (in many instances the area of damaged cells which cause seizures may be no bigger than the point of a pin); vascular disorders (stroke); liver disease; alteration in blood sugar; vitamin deficiencies, and dehydration. Anything that causes a sudden decrease in the flow of blood to the head may be a cause for seizures. Cardiac arrest, low blood pressure, hypertension, arteriosclerosis, sinus sensitivity, DPT shots and artificial sweeteners have been identified as contributing factors to the cause of seizures.

The leading cause of epilepsy for adults is automobile accidents. The leading cause for children is birth trauma. The leading cause for those over 65 is strokes.

Classification

Epilepsy may show itself in a number of ways. The World Health Organization lists over 50 variations of seizures in their "Dictionary of Epilepsy." The kind of seizure a person has is determined by where the electrical disturbance in the brain begins, where it spreads, and how fast it spreads. Sometimes a person tends to have only one kind of seizure, but often more than one type is experienced. The type of epilepsy one has is usually classified by type of seizure. Most people are familiar with the old terminology of three classifications of epilepsy: grand mal ("big illness"), petit mal ("little illness"), and psychomotor (temporal lobe).

A new classification system has been devised, referred to as the International Classification System. Types of epilepsy have been divided into four groups:

I. PARTIAL SEIZURES (affecting only part of the brain)

A. *Simple Partial Seizures* (conscious and aware)

    1. Motor symptoms (muscle, Jacksonian)
    2. Sensory symptoms (touch, taste, sight, smell, hearing)
    3. Autonomic symptoms (internal organs, headache)
    4. Compound forms

B. *Complex Partial Seizures* (some loss of consciousness)

    1. Consciousness impairment only
    2. Cognitive (thought)
    3. Affective (mood, emotions)
    4. Psychosensory (illusions, hallucinations)
    5. Psychomotor (abnormal behavior)
    6. Compound forms

C. *Partial Seizures Secondarily Generalized* (begins as a partial seizure, then becomes generalized)

II. GENERALIZED SEIZURES (affecting the entire brain; loss of consciousness)

    1. Absence (petit mal)
    2. Myoclonus (contractions of major muscles)
    3. Tonic (muscles rigid)
    4. Clonic (jerking movements)
    5. Tonic Clonic (grand mal)
    6. Atonic (loss of muscle tone—person falls down)
    7. Akinetic (loss of movement—person drops things)

III. UNILATERAL SEIZURES (involving one hemisphere, or half, of the brain, affecting one side of the body)

IV. UNCLASSIFIED SEIZURES (because of incomplete information, these cannot be put into a category)

The most common types of seizures from the International Classification System are:

PARTIAL SEIZURES (affecting part of the brain)

a. Simple Partial (conscious and aware)
b. Complex Partial (some loss of consciousness)

GENERALIZED SEIZURES (affecting the entire brain)

a. Tonic Clonic (loss of consciousness)
b. Absence (loss of consciousness for a few seconds)

Auras

Many people who have partial seizures experience a warning or "aura," often described only as a hard-to-explain feeling, before their seizures begin. Hippocrates named the aura, which is a Greek word meaning "breeze." The aura may be a funny feeling in the stomach, a sense of fear, an unusual sound, such as ringing in the ears, or a visual sensation. Sometimes the aura is explained as a strange smell or a vague feeling that something is wrong. The aura is actually a simple partial seizure. Many people have the same aura every time before a seizure. Some have the aura only occasionally. A true generalized seizure is not preceded by an aura.

Seizures

There are many other types of seizures. In fact, every person experiences a unique seizure. Here I will describe some of the most common types.

When the seizure affects movement, it may consist of a spasm, the rhythmic jerking of a limb or, as seen in the *Jacksonian seizure* type, it may begin in a certain area of the body and spread ("march") in an orderly manner involving adjacent muscles. It is named after Hughlings Jackson, an English doctor who made a detailed study of seizures that occurred in his wife. An example of this type of seizure might begin with jerking in the thumb, spread to the fingers, then advance to the wrist, up the forearm to the upper arm and finally to the face. This is one of the simple partial seizures. Sometimes the spasms spread throughout the whole body, resulting in a grand mal seizure (a secondarily generalized seizure).

If the simple partial seizure affects sensation, the person may experience tingling in one part of the body or other unfamiliar feelings. Others may smell things, see flashes of light, or hear sounds that are not really there.

Autonomic seizures (a type of simple partial seizure) affect the autonomic nervous system, which controls involuntary body functions such as digestion and heartbeat. These seizures do not involve the whole brain, nor do they produce unconsciousness. Their symptoms are headaches that occur repeatedly without apparent cause, stomach aches, nausea, vomiting, or fever. Since these symptoms occur in many other conditions, only a thorough physical examination can show whether they are caused by epilepsy.

The *psychomotor seizure,* sometimes called *temporal lobe epilepsy,* is one of the complex partial seizures. It usually arises from one of the temporal lobe areas of the brain, just above the ears. The temporal lobe plays a crucial role in controlling memory, thought and behavior. During a psychomotor seizure the individual's awareness or responsiveness is affected, and she or he is in a sort of dream state. Afterward, the person remembers little or nothing of what happened during the attack.

Commonly this seizure consists of two stages (actually two seizures). There may first be an aura—a strange sensation (a small seizure). The person is then immobile for about ten seconds. This is followed by a period during which the individual begins some purposeless, repetitive action or motion called an *automatism.* An automatism may consist of fidgeting, picking at or removing one's clothes, stroking the hair, lip-smacking or chewing motions, walking about aimlessly, repeating short, senseless phrases over and over, or any type of repetitive or inappropriate action.

The "automatic" behavior in an automatism varies from person to person. The person having the psychomotor seizure often vigorously resists any help offered during the attack. Screaming or using force to try to stop a person having a psychomotor seizure will sometimes make the seizure more intense.

A complex partial seizure usually lasts less than five minutes, however there is often confusion after the seizure. This *postictal confusion* (ictal meaning seizure) is sometimes referred to as *Todd's phenomena,* an aura after a seizure.

Some complex partial seizures may consist of a "dreamy state." During this dreamy state the person may feel like something has happened before (sometimes such a feeling is called by its French name, déjà vu); or he or she may feel unfamiliar in a known place (jamais vu), or he or she may experience an attack where music is heard, vivid scenes are recalled, or tastes or smells are perceived. People having complex partial seizures in public are often mistaken for being drunk or on drugs. Sometimes a psychomotor seizure progresses into a tonic clonic (grand mal) seizure. This is called a secondarily generalized convulsion.

Complex partial seizures are the most difficult seizures to control with medicine; medication often is less than 50% effective.

Complex partial seizures are experienced mostly by adults.

The *absence* (petit mal) seizure is a generalized seizure, affecting the entire brain. This type of seizure most often affects children, and is characterized by staring spells or a momentary lapse of consciousness (often mistaken for daydreaming or inattentiveness). The attack is sudden and without warning, lasting only a few seconds. Activity abruptly stops and a momentary trance-like state occurs. Then, as suddenly as it comes, the trance-like state disappears, and the individual recovers immediately.

Not every absence seizure is alike. Some involve a twitching or rhythmic movement of the facial muscles or head or arms, while others involve rapid eye blinking or rolling the eyes upward. Muscles may sharply contract, or muscle control may be reduced. There may be a blank stare or blank look into an observer's eyes (some call these "hate looks"). The person may be inattentive or "spacey" (especially if it is in the middle of other activities). The person may fail to answer when his or her name is spoken, and may be unresponsive to the surroundings. The individual may be unaware that there has been a lapse of consciousness. As a result, the person usually continues his or her activities following the seizure as if nothing had happened.

Absence seizures often go unnoticed by family, friends and school personnel. If a child is having absence seizures (blanking out for a few seconds) at school, he or she may miss part of what the teacher is saying. Absence seizures may occur as frequently as 200 – 300 times a day. Absence seizures usually disappear by age 20. Many adults who think they are having absence seizures may be experiencing partial seizures, and may be taking incorrect medication.

In infants there may be massive myoclonic episodes that have been termed *infantile spasms*. These usually occur many times a day and tend to be associated with brain damage and mental retardation. In this type of seizure there is a sudden muscular contraction by which the head is flexed, the arms extended and the legs drawn up. This syndrome is often confused with colic or other gastro-intestinal disturbances before their convulsive nature is recognized.

A *unilateral seizure* is an attack which sometimes occurs during infancy. With this type of seizure only one side of the body is affected. Facial muscles, arm muscles, or leg muscles on one side twitch violently, while those on the other side remain under control. The person is usually conscious during a unilateral seizure.

Tonic clonic (grand mal) seizures are the type of seizures most people are familiar with and which they associate with epilepsy. A tonic clonic seizure is a type of generalized seizure.

This is a violent major attack where the person suddenly loses consciousness. The person often falls to the ground and experiences a sudden sharp stiffening of the muscles. He or she may give a sharp cry as air is forced through the voice box. This is the tonic (stiffening) phase. The tonic rigidity soon passes and is replaced by a rapid jerking of all parts of the body. The person thrashes the arms and legs about, the jaw jerks and the tongue may be bitten. This is the clonic phase. The seizure is often accompanied by irregular or interrupted breathing and the individual may turn blue for a short period of time. There may be some drooling or frothing of saliva, as well as involuntary loss of urine or stool.

A tonic clonic seizure may last from less than a minute up to half an hour or more. The seizure may occur many times a day or as infrequently as once in several years. The attacks may be mostly during sleep, but are usually spread throughout the entire 24 hours. Following the seizure, the individual may feel tired, confused, weak, nauseated, restless or irritable for some time. Some individuals require a short nap, while others fall into deep sleep for several hours. Many people need a lot of sleep for several days afterward. Rarely does a person return immediately to normal activity.

Very rarely, a tonic clonic seizure can turn into a dangerous form of attack called *status epilepticus*. In this form the storm in the brain does not quiet down. One seizure follows another. If this continues for over 10 minutes and no medical assistance is provided, death can occur.

Medication is effective in controlling tonic clonic (grand mal) seizures approximately 80% of the time. Valium is effective for about 40 minutes in stopping an uncontrolled seizure. It is sometimes inserted in the rectum of a child whose life may be in danger because of status epilepticus.

The tonic clonic (generalized) seizure which follows a complex partial or simple partial seizure is a secondarily generalized seizure.

It is rare for a person to have more than one major type of epilepsy. Since most people have only one type of epilepsy, monotherapy (one drug) is most effective for most people. Careful observation of the beginning of each seizure is important. This information helps the physician diagnose and to prescribe the medication which will be most effective. If the seizure begins as a partial, medicine for generalized tonic clonic seizures is probably inappropriate. Talk with your prescribing physician if you have questions about your medication.

Many people believe they have more than one type of epilepsy because a seizure begins as a partial seizure and progresses (spreads) to a generalized seizure. These people are, in fact, experiencing more than one type of seizure. However, they usually have only one type of epilepsy, and this is determined by the *focus*. The focus is the spot in the brain where there is damage and is where the seizure activity begins.

Seizure Emergency Checklist

While a person is experiencing a seizure, there is actually nothing you can do to stop the seizure, so stay calm and follow this guide.

1. Do not restrain—it can make the seizure more severe.

2. Stay nearby.

3. Speak kindly.

4. If the person is moving around, remove dangerous, sharp or hot objects from the area.

5. Stand behind the person and gently guide him or her away from danger.

6. If the person shakes or falls, turn the head or whole body to the side so that saliva can drain from the mouth.

7. Force nothing between the teeth. The outdated practice of putting

an object in the mouth to prevent the person from swallowing the tongue is not appropriate. The tongue cannot be swallowed. A hard object can increase the damage to the tongue from biting. A soft object can become lodged in the throat, causing suffocation.

I believe these guidelines should be known by everyone, not just the families and friends of those with epilepsy. More than once, I have had well-meaning people call an ambulance for me, not knowing that it is unnecessary unless the seizure lasts longer than 10 minutes. Coming out of a seizure with paramedics standing over me added to the shock and embarrassment as I gradually regained consciousness, trying to realize where I was and what had happened. The bills (several hundred dollars) were an added shock since my income was at a poverty level.

I have a scar on my tongue because some observers put a hard object across my tongue while I was having a grand mal seizure. They were recalling old advice, and were trying to protect me from biting or swallowing my tongue.

----

[1]*Epilepsy, Breaking Down the Walls of Misunderstanding,* pamphlet, Abbott Laboratories.

[2]*Facts and Figures on the Epilepsies,* pamphlet, Epilepsy Society of America, p.5.

Chapter 3

Neurofeedback: Learn to Control Your Brain Waves with EEG Biofeedback

*"You cannot step into the same river twice.
The new water is always rushing in."*

—*Greek philosopher Heraclitus*

The atoms in the body and brain are like the new water always rushing into the river. 98% of the atoms in your body were not there a year ago. You can have some control over the new atoms in your body as well as in shaping the old patterns in the brain, by using biofeedback.

Learning to control the electrical activity of your brain is a very promising avenue to explore if you are ready to try a new approach to the treatment of epilepsy. For many people it is possible to reduce or eliminate seizures through EEG (electroencephalograph) biofeedback training. It is a learning strategy that helps you to change your brain wave activity. Think of it as physical therapy for the brain. However, this takes willpower, time and persistence.

We have billions of brain cells, but we only use a small portion of those cells. Many are simply idle. People with epilepsy have brains that continuously misfire (not just during seizures), which shows up in EEG's and allows neurologists to make a diagnosis. This continuous misfiring may only involve a few brain cells, the area of misfiring no bigger than the point of a pin. The brain cells surrounding the misfiring or damaged cells are sometimes activated to misfire as well, resulting in a seizure.

Since the 1970's researchers have demonstrated in over 50 controlled studies that a special form of brain wave biofeedback—now called "neurofeedback"—safely and effectively trains the brain to stabilize its activity, allowing medication to be cautiously reduced (with your physician's supervision) or in some cases eliminated altogether. The treatment has been used successfully with all types of seizure disorder. It works with adults and children alike. Some serious disorders require booster sessions; however, often the effects are permanent,

Neurofeedback treatment involves performing two or more 30-minute sessions per week, after a preliminary evaluation to determine the protocol. The evaluation involves some or all of the following: an EEG "brain map" or *Quantitative EEG,* a neuro-detailed history, a TOVA test (Test of Variables of Attention, often used for Attention Deficit Disorder [ADD] or Attention Deficit Hyperactivity Disorder [ADHD] testing), and a baseline EEG.

In training sessions, special computerized biofeedback instrumentation detects and displays the brain waves generated by the seizure disorder on a computer screen. The computer program allows for simultaneous inhibition of slow wave (4 – 7 Hz) and very fast wave (22 – 30 Hz) and reinforcement of mid-range frequencies (12 – 15 Hz or 15 – 18 Hz). Patients are then taught how to modify their brain waves to prevent seizures, by gradually shaping the EEG to decrease amplitude of slow brain wave activity associated with seizures. Much of the learning takes place simply with practice while receiving positive reinforcement from the computer. After enough training sessions (the number varies between individuals) the aura rate goes down and so does the seizure rate. (EEG biofeedback training is also very effective for children with ADD and ADHD.)

No one knows exactly what occurs as we learn to "normalize" the brain wave activity (produce EEG patterns which don't trigger seizures). But it works.

Understanding Biofeedback

Biofeedback, short for biological feedback, is basically the monitoring of internal body states. You learn this by watching and listening to sensitive instruments that mirror psychophysiological processes of which you are not normally aware. An electronic instrument detects, amplifies, then gives you immediate information (feedback) about your own biological or physiological conditions, such as: brain wave activity (EEG), muscle tension (EMG) or skin temperature. This instantaneous feedback guides you as you create appropriate psychological or physical changes, becoming more in touch with your mind and body.

Biofeedback instruments have meters, lights, computer displays and sounds, which relay information to you, telling the mind what the body is doing. The information guides you as you create appropriate psychological and physical change, bringing mind and body under control. The body responds to and can be directed by the mind. The body and mind interact, and are really inseparable. A good example of this is when you decide to wiggle the thumb on your right hand. Your brain sends many signals, the proper nerves and muscles respond, and you wiggle your right thumb within a fraction of a second.

You have actually been using biofeedback all your life—without electrical equipment. You do this by looking in a mirror, weighing yourself, taking your temperature, learning to play a musical instrument, learning to ride a bike or to play basketball.

Imagine that you are learning to play basketball. You throw the ball, and receive information back from the basket by seeing whether the ball went through the basket or not. If it did not, you notice where the ball landed. This is the feedback of information you use to improve your second shot. You continually try different techniques for throwing the ball. You move to the left, and then move to the right, throw the ball a little harder, etc., until the ball goes through the basket. As you practice you become more aware and gain control. You finally reach your goal, a basket.

Feedback of information to the learner makes learning possible, whether learning to talk, walk, ride a bicycle, read, play a musical instrument or tell a good joke. Without feedback of information learning is impossible. Imagine trying to learn to get the ball in the basket while blindfolded.

Now imagine trying to learn to control your brain waves. You cannot feel, see, hear or in any way directly detect the electrical activity of your brain. You have a general idea of how your brain is operating; however, you lack awareness of your intricate brain activity and therefore you lack direct control. Imagine, however, that you are connected to an instrument which is designed to detect the electrical activity of the brain, and to convert the activity into meaningful information which you can hear or see—brain wave feedback. Using the information from the feedback machine as a guide, you could learn to control your brain waves in the same way that information from the basket guides you while learning to throw the basketball.

Biofeedback training starts out with your brain waves totally uncontrolled. You gradually gain control over functions which you thought were involuntary, and eventually, the control becomes automatic. Some of this learning is by "passive volition," which requires that you are aware of your task, but you are not trying too hard. A phrase often used for this is "letting it happen."

Biofeedback instruments make it much easier for you to use your mind to control both physical (physiological) and mental (psychological) functions. The instrument tells the mind what the body is doing; then your complex mental processes are directed to create change in your physiological functioning. The conscious mind knows or feels that a certain effect is desired, but needs to practice and experiment until the final result is what you had imagined.

Neurofeedback

There are many types of biofeedback training. The method which is usually used for epilepsy therapy is neurofeedback (brain wave feedback) training, using an instrument called the EEG, short for electroencephalograph. The EEG instrument measures the speed (frequency) and intensity (amplitude) of the brain waves and "feeds back" the information to the trainee, visually (by watching a computer screen with a meter, graph or lights) and aurally (by listening to a sound). Instruments which measure both the frequency and amplitude of the brain waves are the most helpful for learning to control seizures.

The human brain produces continuous electrical signals. The strength or amplitude of these signals is so small that it is measured in microvolts, or millionths of a volt. The signals are picked up by electrodes or sensors touching the surface of the head and then amplified hundreds of times.

The most common technique involves the therapist parting the trainee's hair, and, for accuracy, pasting one or two tiny flat discs (electrodes) onto the scalp and one to an ear. These discs pick up the electrical current from the brain. The electrode wire then carries the current to the biofeedback instrument to be read. The computer-based instrumentation records the raw EEG, all brain wave activity at the site of the sensor. The computer program separates the raw EEG into frequency bands and displays them separately. The patient uses this display to learn to inhibit slow wave activity (4 – 7 or 2 – 7 Hz) and excessive fast wave activity (22 – 30 Hz) while simultaneously reinforcing the midrange frequencies (12 – 15 or 15 – 18 Hz). When the EEG is used for diagnostic purposes, a different procedure is used; many electrodes are placed at certain points all over the head.

Brain Waves

The neurons in the brain are constantly firing, producing a mixture of electrical activity, some slow, some moderate, and some fast in frequency. This electrical activity or brain wave activity is divided into frequency bands with a computer-based system to describe how fast or slow the electrical activity is occurring. Even though there will be a mixture of all frequencies happening simultaneously, there will be more of one frequency band at any one time (the dominant frequency).

When looking at an encephalogram (the brain wave activity recorded on paper), frequency is displayed horizontally. The faster frequencies will appear narrower, and the slower frequencies will be wider. Amplitude (strength of the wave) is displayed vertically. High amplitude activity will look taller and lower amplitude activity will look shorter. Slower frequencies tend to have higher peaks (amplitude).

The brain waves are divided into frequency "bands," using Greek letters for naming them. The term "Hertz," (Hz) means frequency or cycles per second. The higher the numbers, the faster the electrical activity of the brain.

Gamma: 24 Hz and above

Sometimes referred to as high beta.

Produced during intense concentration or anxiety.

If there is also high amplitude, this usually indicates excessive effort.

With neurofeedback, this also reflects excess muscle tension.

Beta: 15 – 18 Hz

Produced during focused attention. Many people with head trauma or depression don't produce as much beta as others.

SMR (Sensorimotor Rhythm): 12 – 15 Hz

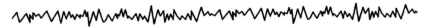

Sometimes referred to as low beta. A state of relaxed concentration. Also produced in sleep while dreaming, and called REM, short for Rapid Eye Movement.

Often used for seizure control and hyperactivity.

M.B. Sterman, Ph.D., a pioneer in neurofeedback for the treatment of epilepsy, only trained the sensorimotor cortex in his research. The rhythm is named for its location. All brain waves can be produced in any part of the brain.

Alpha: 8 – 12 Hz

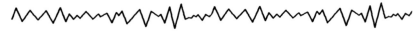

Associated with general relaxation and meditation.

Theta: 4 – 7 Hz

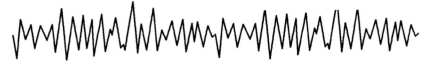

Associated with drowsiness, inattention, daydreaming, creativity, and deep meditation. Many people who have experienced head trauma, and have been diagnosed with epilepsy, ADD or ADHD produce an abundance of 4 – 7 Hz activity.

Delta: .05 – 3 Hz

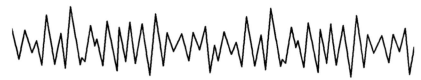

Produced in deep dreamless sleep.

No specific frequency band is "good" or "bad," and the brain needs to operate predominantly in different bands at different times for different tasks. However, sometimes the brain seems to be like a train off its track (i.e., there may be an abundance of theta activity and not enough beta activity, resulting in seizures or involuntary body movement, inattention or memory problems). Neurofeedback training can help the brain to get back on track.

Brain wave activity is rather complex, and may exhibit several frequencies simultaneously at any given instant. Many people who have seizures produce a combination of beta and alpha brain waves, with frequent abnormal bursts of theta. During their normal day-to-day activities and during sleep, their EEG's will read abnormal. People who have complex partial (psychomotor) seizures usually have occasional "spikes," or bursts, of high amplitude waves from one of the temporal lobes. Those who have absence (petit mal) seizures usually have occasional discharges in a pattern called the three-second spike-and-wave. During a seizure, the spike-and-wave discharge is very rhythmical and continuous.

EEG's of people with epilepsy look something like this:

Spike-and-slow-wave discharge

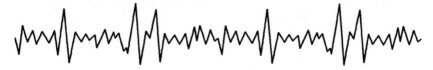

Three-second spike-and-wave characteristic of Absence (Petit Mal)

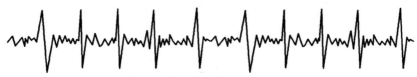

Tonic Clonic discharge during seizure

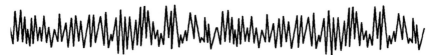

For comparison, the EEG of a person without epilepsy would look something like this:

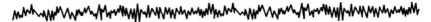

Since slower frequencies tend to be accompanied by high amplitude peaks, relaxing, "letting go" and meditating are not helpful for most people *during the aura* (the beginning of a seizure). Producing slow brain waves with high amplitude peaks may encourage seizures for some people. Paradoxically, meditating and relaxing (except at the onset of a seizure) once a day for 20 minutes tends to reduce the seizure threshold. Allowing the brain and body to completely relax once a day seems to take the place of having a seizure.

Neurofeedback Research

M. B. Sterman, Ph.D., while chief of neuropsychology research at the Veteran's Administration Hospital in Sepulveda, California, was the first researcher to discover that brain wave training could affect epileptic seizures. Dating back to the 1970's, he and his colleagues had demonstrated that cats could be conditioned to control their brain wave patterns by rewarding them with food each time they would produce a certain type of brain wave pattern.

Some cats were taught to increase the percentage of 12 – 15 Hz brain wave rhythm.[1] Sterman called this pattern the sensorimotor rhythm (SMR) because the electrodes were over an area of the brain (approximately 1 to 2 inches above the ear at the temple) called the sensorimotor cortex.

About that time, NASA approached Sterman because of a problem they were having; their rocket fuel appeared to be inducing seizures in their personnel on the test range. While testing the hydrocarbon fuel for its convulsive effects on the nervous system, Sterman accidentally discovered that two of the five cats who were trained to produce SMR also gained the ability to delay convulsions.[2] He decided to explore the possibility that humans, too, could decrease seizure activity by learning to produce SMR. During many months of training Sterman found that seizure activity indeed decreased in four human subjects as they learned to produce SMR.

In a later study, in order to establish the validity of the EEG training technique, Sterman and MacDonald conducted a controlled study. In this study, "yoked controls" were used, where the feedback signal to the patient, unbeknownst to him or her, was periodically reversed from another patient. Other controlled studies were done at a later date.

Researchers in other laboratories and clinics have found that through neurofeedback, training subjects may experience reductions and severity of seizures. Some subjects have been able to reduce medication as well, with their physician's guidance.

One of these researchers, Judith Green, Ph.D., conducted a study at the Menninger Foundation in Topeka, Kansas. She worked with four people who had epilepsy.[3] Two subjects received alpha feedback (10 – 13 Hz) and two received beta feedback (15 – 20 Hz). One trainee receiving beta feedback could produce beta when she created in her mind a "strong" bright image of the sun. Several months after training, she reported she could block seizures if there was time during the aura. Both beta trainees experienced a reduction in seizures.

Whitsett, Lubar, et al, studied eight severely epileptic patients.[4] Training was done in three phases. All-night recordings were obtained at the end of each conditioning phase. Their findings showed that EEG biofeedback might produce changes in the sleep EEG that are related to seizure evidence.

Wyler, et al, studied 23 patients who had severe epileptic seizures.[5] The aim of their study was to reinforce the individual's 18 Hz activity over the scalp approximation of abnormal brain wave activity. They reported that many of their patients showed a reduction in seizure activity.

Research by Bruner, Tansey and Chinisci has shown that many people who have epilepsy trained to produce a specific frequency (some produced 12 Hz, others 13 Hz, others 14 Hz) reported a reduction in seizures.[6] Electrode placement for their training was the top of the head. Bruner, et al, believe relaxation is a contributing factor in seizure reduction.

The most extensive research in EEG training for epilepsy has shown that training for 12 – 14 Hz (SMR) or 15 – 18 Hz (beta) while inhibiting 4 – 7 Hz abnormal spike and wave activity is most effective for reducing or preventing seizures. This means the brain will be operating at a "moderate" tempo, with no sudden breaks or slowing down. This involves concentrating or focusing with the eyes open and the body relaxed. Some individuals practicing this type of biofeedback have described it as: "physical therapy with the brain," "mental calisthenics," "having fun," "making a circuit bypass," "telling the brain to 'do it'," "hard work," and "relaxing and feeling positive energy." No matter what feelings or thoughts accompany the training, the common pattern for success is to give a message or cue to oneself, then to relax and let it happen (passive volition).

Putting It into Practice

With practice, producing the desired brain wave activity becomes easier, more natural, and eventually automatic. Some people notice changes in seizure activity after only a few sessions; however, it usually takes many months before there is a significant lessening of the number and severity of seizures.

The length of time usually required to achieve control is the main drawback to this treatment. It can take from 80 – 100 training sessions, which is much longer than biofeedback training for other problems. Most insurance companies and HMO's are unaware of the research and benefits, so the training can be expensive. Persistence and motivation are important for the learner. When positive results are seen, they may be dramatic. In addition to reductions in the number and severity of seizures, cognitive skills may improve, there may be a gradual reduction of medication (under the active supervision of the prescribing physician) and/or a normalization of the EEG. It is extremely important to follow the advice of a physician as training proceeds.

Visualization and direction is a part of the training sessions. Since, in a person with epilepsy, a group of brain cells may be damaged or misfiring, during sessions, you may want to visualize having surrounding brain cells do the work of the damaged cells, or direct new dendrites to send signals between brain cells in a different way.

There are side-benefits of EEG training. The concentration which is necessary to gain control over the brain wave activity tends to inhibit the bursts of undesirable slow spike-and-wave activity. Training promotes relaxation, which in turn also affects the number of seizures related to stress. Keeping records of seizures and circumstances surrounding each seizure increases awareness of situations which trigger seizures, so the person can avoid those situations.

Even though brain cells die each day, we still have plenty to last a lifetime. The average person uses approximately 10% of their brain cells. However, new dendrites, the connections which send signals between brain cells, are continually being born, no matter what our age. As we learn new things (exercise the brain), more and more new dendrites are formed. This is the best prevention for aging and memory loss as well as for healing—especially nervous system and brain disorders such as epilepsy.

My Own Healing Path

Learning self-regulation and awareness by controlling the electrical activity of my brain through a combination of SMR (12 – 15 Hz) training and meditation was helpful for me. The majority of my biofeedback training was aimed at producing SMR. Gaining control over brain wave activity is very subtle and can be lengthy. It took several training sessions before I was able to consciously change my brain wave activity for brief periods of time. I gradually learned by trial and error how to consciously regulate my mind and body. Many months of training were necessary for me to feel control of my brain wave activity for any length of time.

I learned that my brain wave activity would change quickly from a very rapid to a very slow pattern, which is typical of people with epilepsy. This is called *hyperpolarized cortical excitability* and is characterized by slow (4 – 7 Hz) brain wave activity which occurs for longer periods of time than in those who don't have epilepsy. The slow activity is followed by periods of faster (alpha and beta) brain wave activity.

My training was done at the Aims Biofeedback Institute, Aims Community College, Greeley, Colorado, under the supervision of Robert Shellenberger, Ph.D., John Turner, Ph.D., and Ron Petersen, with frequent advice from Judith Green, Ph.D.

I practiced three times each week for approximately three years before I was in complete control of my seizures. At the beginning of training my seizure rate was 10 to 15 seizures per month. Progress was not steady. I would have a period of complete control (no seizures), then a regression (one seizure or more).

Biofeedback training is a unique experience. Suggestions from others may be helpful, although the thoughts and feelings which produce certain types of brain waves for one person may produce different brain wave patterns for another.

I will share with you my thoughts and feelings while practicing neurofeedback as well as I can in words. My first and main goal in training was to produce 12 – 15 Hz low amplitude (SMR) brain waves. To accomplish this, I found that I needed to concentrate on something very intently, with my eyes open, such as doing multiplication, thinking of a sequence or pattern of numbers, visualizing certain scenes, or imagining that I was reading and hearing some words or music. This concentration created the 12 – 15 Hz brain waves, although it was tiring and I could only do it for a short time. There were still occasional high amplitude spikes in my EEG, and I couldn't seem to eliminate them.

I finally discovered that if I consciously relaxed, especially my throat and shoulder muscles, while breathing deeply, still concentrating very intently on a subject in my mind, I would produce SMR. All of this needed to be done without too much effort!

Another feeling and image I used was that the center of my body was very alert and full of energy, which I visualized as white light going up my spine to the top of my head. The outside of my body was relaxed; my shoulders, arms and jaw were dropped downward. My jaw would be centered with my tongue in the bottom of my mouth, heavy and relaxed. This awareness showed me something very important; it is possible to be relaxed even while concentrating intently! The mind can be alert and active while the body is relaxed. This is sometimes called "letting it happen" or *passive volition* and is helpful in all types of biofeedback training as well as relaxation, meditation (and with everything we do).

Another method which was very helpful for me was to imagine and concentrate on a light rhythmic tune at the top of my head, sometimes repeating syllables silently with the tune. I had a light-hearted feeling while doing this, yet I was very much aware of what I was concentrating on. All of my SMR training was done with my eyes open.

After learning to produce SMR, I began to practice meditation with biofeedback equipment. The alpha training was to confirm what was occurring. I found that by taking time to relax and meditate for 15 minutes twice each day, I would seldom have seizures. I believe the reason for the reduction in seizures was because my brain and nervous system needed time to rest, time for my brain to produce slow brain waves. At times when I was going in "high gear" for too long, not stopping to rest or meditate, I would be more likely to have a seizure. Meditation is discussed more thoroughly in Chapter 4.

My different steps to achieve SMR and alpha were the following:

ALPHA (8 – 12 Hz)	SMR (12 – 15 Hz)
Eyes closed	Eyes open
Slow, deep breathing	Slow, deep breathing
Muscles relaxed	Muscles relaxed
Concentrating on one syllable or object for a short time	Continuous alert concentration
Forgetting everything	
Listening quietly	

I gradually learned to switch my mode of brain wave activity at will after both SMR and alpha training. This gave me control of a previous automatic function. Now, when I want to be alert and active, I use the thoughts and feelings which produce SMR. When I want to rest (once or twice each day), I stop and meditate or relax. My goal is moderation in my brain wave activity.

The aura (the feeling or beginning of an upcoming seizure) seldom occurred before I started neurofeedback. My awareness increased with training to the point where a seizure would seldom slip up on me. To stop a seizure I would take a deep breath, fight the seizure, resist the urge to give up, saying to myself, "I am not going to have a seizure!" It would take every bit of energy I could gather for the next few seconds or minutes to block the seizure and redirect my brain wave energy. This concentration, determination, adrenaline and extra oxygen to my brain would normalize neuronal activity and abort the seizure.

The final result of the EEG biofeedback (neurofeedback) training was that the helpful brain wave pattern became automatic. There are now no seizures to stop when I daily visualize or feel the SMR brain wave pattern.

If you have auras before seizures so that you know when a seizure is coming on, why not try stopping your next one, whether you've had biofeedback training or not? Say to yourself, "I am going to stop this seizure!" Take a deep breath, resist the urge to give in. Focus on your surroundings. (For different breathing procedures refer to Chapter Four of this book.) Use every bit of energy you can gather for the next few seconds or minutes. If you always go into a seizure without warning, ask for help from those who might be with you. Tell them that the instant they see you beginning to have a seizure, they should say something like, "You're going to stop this seizure. You can do it."

It takes energy, willpower, desire and determination to stop a seizure. If you stop one after many tries, be proud of yourself. This will be proof that it can be done. Then ask yourself, "If I can stop one seizure, what's keeping me from stopping or eliminating more seizures?"

Remember that your brain may be producing abnormal spike-and-wave activity 24 hours a day every day, but you don't have seizures 24 hours every day.

The brain is a marvelous mechanical organ which orchestrates everything that goes on in your body, consciously, subconsciously or automatically. The mind is not the same thing as the brain. You are a soul or spirit living in your body, the brain included, for the time being.

---

[1] Maurice B. Sterman, *Neurophysiologic and Clinical Studies of Sensorimotor Cortex, EEG Feedback Training: Some Effects on Epilepsy,* Seminars in Psychiatry (1974): pp. 507-525.

[2] Maurice B. Sterman, R.W. Lo Presti, Fairchild, M.D., *Electroencephalographic and Behavioral Studies of Monomethyl Hydrazine Toxicity in the Cat,* Technical Report AMRL-TR-69-3, Air Systems Command, (Wright-Patterson Air Force Base, OH 1969).

[3] Judith A. Green, Ph.D., *Brain-Wave Training for Seizure Reduction in Epilepsy,* dissertation, Union Graduate School (1976).

[4] S.F. Whitsett, J.F. Lubar, Holder, Pamplin and Shabsin, *A Double-Blind Investigation of the Relationship Between Seizure Activity and the Sleep EEG Following EEG Biofeedback Training,* Biofeedback and Self-Regulation (1982).

[5] Fischer-Williams, M.D., Nigel, Ph.E. and Sovine, Ph.D., *A Textbook of Biological Feedback* (New York: Human Sciences Press, 1981): pp. 178-180.

[6] Bruner, Tansey and Chinisci, Presentation, Biofeedback Society of America Convention (Denver, CO, 1983).

Chapter 4

Stress: Enough is Enough!

Raise Your Seizure Threshold to Prevent Seizures

Stress can lead to drastic changes in the chemistry of the body; chemical changes can be a cause of seizures. Although this concept is not new, it is underrated medically.

Stress can be caused by overwork, inactivity, trying to achieve perfection, dissatisfaction with others, worry, fear, anger, not enough sleep, eating too much of the wrong foods, not eating often enough, relationship differences, too much to do in too little time, not enough money, tense situations in work or family, etc., etc. This list could go on and on and fill an entire book, but I'm sure you get the picture. Everyone has a weakness or vulnerability to stress.

When these stressors aggravate us to a certain point (our threshold), the central nervous system says, "Enough is enough!" One person might get a tension headache, another a backache, another heartburn, someone else a migraine, another person's arthritis pain might get worse. For those of us who are vulnerable to seizures, we might have a seizure.

None of these disorders are imaginary, nor are they a sign of failure. As human beings we all have certain physical, emotional and psychological characteristics. The person with epilepsy is vulnerable to seizures because of certain misfirings of neurons in the brain. They may be so subtle that an EEG won't pick them up (*idiopathic epilepsy*) or they may be very obvious. These abnormal brain wave patterns may be from trauma (an injury) or we may have simply been born that way. Often the cause is unknown.

The important thing is that we don't have seizures 24 hours a day, every day. What is happening physically and psychologically the few hours, days or weeks before a seizure determines our *seizure threshold*; that point when the central nervous system says, "Enough is enough!"

Stress seemed to be responsible for triggering many seizures for me. At times I would be unaware of the stress until later; then I would try to recall what the cause of the seizure could have been. Almost every time I had been either hurrying, worrying, excited, bored, hungry, fearful or tired (usually a combination of any of these things). For instance, the beginning of a new class, whether I would be teaching or attending as a student, would be a signal to watch for a seizure. Traveling grew to be something I would dread rather than look forward to since it would be a likely time for a seizure to occur. Since skipping meals would sometimes cause a seizure, that meant that I needed to have a fairly neat, organized lifestyle.

The cycle of stress and seizures needed to be broken, and one way was to learn to relax more easily and more often. The EEG biofeedback training made it possible for me to stop many seizures, but there were still times when my mind would be too busy with things at hand, and I would forget to produce the necessary brain wave activity.

I found it was helpful to practice some methods of relaxation every day, varying the methods at different times. Some of these methods are: deep breathing, yoga asanas (postures), meditation, progressive relaxation, autogenic phrases, visualization, imagery and affirmations. I will describe each of these methods so you can understand them; then you can practice those which you think will help you to relax more easily.

Any method of relaxation will help to combat the popularly labeled "fight-or-flight" response which causes many harmful effects on our bodies. The fight-or-flight response is an inborn reaction which was very necessary and helpful for our ancestors to survive. Millions of years ago, when a person was faced with stress, he or she would automatically have an increase in blood pressure, heart beat, rate of breathing, blood flow to the muscles, and metabolism, preparing them to fight the attacker or run away. In prehistoric times the use of the fight-or-flight response could mean the difference between life and death.

Our present society also provokes plenty of stress, anxiety and fear which trigger this inborn fight-or-flight response. However, today it is often brought on by situations that require behavioral adjustments where one stays put and in control of one's self. When used inappropriately, which is most of the time, the fight-or-flight response may lead to nervous disease and death. I have noticed that many people with epilepsy are very sensitive. This sensitivity is wonderful, but it can also be an extra burden for the nervous system during times of stress.

You may have already experienced the effects of stress on seizures. Since epilepsy is a disorder of the central nervous system, it would seem logical to assume that stress has an effect on epilepsy. This assumption is correct; 80 – 90% of seizures are caused by stress or excitement. You will need to experiment, using a trial-and-error formula, to determine what type of stress reduction works best for you.

Deep Breathing

Deep breathing is probably the most common and the most beneficial of all relaxation techniques. It can be done anywhere, at any time, and can be combined with other types of stress management.

The simplest exercise for deep breathing is known by many names. Some of these are: abdominal breathing, diaphragmatic breathing, balloon breath, and complete breath.

You can be sitting, standing or lying on your back for deep breathing. Imagine your lungs are divided into thirds, with the bottom third going as low as the abdomen. Your hands are laid on the diaphragm with the middle fingers touching. The little fingers will be at the waist. As you inhale slowly, fill the abdomen (lower third of the lungs) first, feeling it expand. Let the hands rise and separate. Imagine your lungs are filling as a balloon. Next, fill the middle section of the lungs, and finally fill the top third with the healthful, energy-giving oxygen. Exhale slowly and smoothly, starting with the chest or top third, then the middle section, and finally the abdomen as you finish the exhalation. Gently press down with the hands to help get all the carbon dioxide from the lungs.

These sections of your lungs will each be contracting as the carbon dioxide slowly leaves the body—just like a balloon would get smaller as it loses the air it has been holding. Exhaling should be done slowly and through the nostrils. You may find that you have a tendency to contract the abdomen as you inhale rather than expanding it; if so, you will need to concentrate on doing it correctly. It is sometimes helpful to count slowly to yourself during each inhalation and exhalation. At first, use the same amount of time for both inhalation and exhalation, i.e., four counts as you inhale, four counts as you exhale. As you get more accomplished, try to take longer with the exhalation than with the inhalation. The counting for this could be: four counts while inhaling, hold the breath for four counts, then exhale to a count of eight.

Another way to accomplish this is to inhale fully, then exhale slowly as you direct your breath to a burning candle. You can also simply imagine you're blowing out a candle.

One inhalation and one exhalation make up one round of the breathing exercise. Strive for at least three rounds twice daily. This can be done any time you have a few minutes—when you're waiting for someone or waiting in line somewhere, taking a break, before or after meals, before going to sleep, and many more times when you can find the time. The deep breathing exercise can be done without the hands on the diaphragm.

Make sure to exhale slowly. Rapid, consecutive inhalation and exhalation can cause hyperventilation, which can trigger a seizure.

Yoga

Yoga is another way to find some refreshing relaxation. Yoga is an ancient East Indian practice which means "unity of being," or "to yoke." With yoga there is harmony within our physical, mental and spiritual faculties. Through meditation there is a union of our spirit with the Absolute Being or God and the whole universe.

The *asanas* (postures, pronounced awe' suh nuz) are effective not only in the prevention of disease, but also in aiding the cure of existing disease. I will describe a few asanas which you could practice in 10 to 20 minutes. You would benefit from doing even one asana if you are short on time. If you feel that you might benefit from learning more, and would like to spend more time doing asanas, you might want to sign up for a yoga class. There are also many helpful instruction books to guide you, some of which are listed in the back of this book. After you're comfortable doing asanas you may want to try taking a yoga break instead of a coffee break.

There are a few basic guidelines for doing asanas.

1. Wait 1½ – 2 hours after a full meal. Wait at least ½ hour after a light snack.
2. Always stretch but not to the point of pain while doing asanas.
3. Inhale while raising any part of the body, and exhale while lowering the body.
4. Do each asana 1 – 3 times (usually just once).

Neck Exercise—Sitting upright or standing, nod the head forward slowly and hold it a few seconds. Nod to the back and hold it a few seconds. Repeat the forward and backward nodding three times. Nod to the left shoulder and hold it a few seconds. Nod to the right shoulder and hold it a few seconds. Repeat the nodding to each side three times. Slowly roll the head clockwise three times, keeping the face forward and the shoulders still, then reverse. When you've completed this, make fists, tense and raise your shoulders up to your ears, make a face, tensing your facial muscles. Hold for a few seconds then release. This relieves headache, relaxes neck and shoulder tensions.

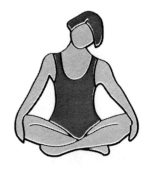

Pelvic Tilt—Lying on the back, bend the knees. Inhale first, then exhale, drawing the stomach muscles back and tightening the buttocks, trying to touch the entire spine to the floor. Hold for a few seconds, then relax. This also can be done standing, with the back against a wall, or sitting in a chair. Simply try to touch the entire spine against the wall or the back of the chair in the same manner. This takes away tension and pain in the lower back, as well as strengthening the muscles of the lower back and abdomen.

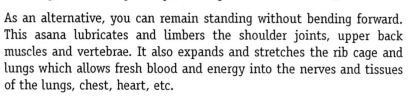

Chest Expansion—From a standing position with legs together, interlock fingers and hands behind the back, straightening the arms, standing erect. Breathe in deeply, raise the arms up and back away from the body, drawing the shoulder blades together. Exhaling slowly, bend forward at the hips, keeping the knees slightly bent and the spine straight. Let the face roll forward, keeping the arms straight. Hold this position, breathing comfortably, then begin to come up slowly, inhaling.

As an alternative, you can remain standing without bending forward. This asana lubricates and limbers the shoulder joints, upper back muscles and vertebrae. It also expands and stretches the rib cage and lungs which allows fresh blood and energy into the nerves and tissues of the lungs, chest, heart, etc.

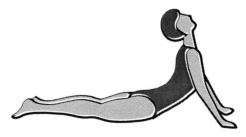

Cobra—Lie on the stomach. Place the hands palms down on the floor beneath the shoulders. The elbows should be bent and close to the body. Inhaling, slowly raise the head and chest from the floor, rolling the head back as far as you can, arching the back. Hold the breath, then exhale while slowly lowering to the floor. Relax and enjoy the effects. This limbers the spine and is excellent for relieving backache.

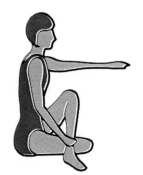

Half Spinal Twist—From a sitting position, wrap the right leg around the body on the floor (or have it straight in front of you on the floor). Cross the left leg over the right leg with the foot flat on the floor as far back as possible. Grasp the left ankle with the right hand or put the right hand on the floor close to your body.

Raise the left arm to shoulder level and twist slowly to the left as you inhale.

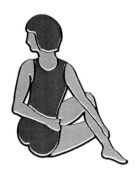

Follow your fingers with your eyes. Bring the left arm behind your back with the elbow bent, striving to touch your navel, or simply put the hand flat on the floor close to your body. Twist the head to the left, looking over the shoulder. Let the shoulders drop down, relaxed. Breathe shallowly as you hold the posture, then straighten the left arm at shoulder level and untwist slowly as you inhale again. Repeat with the other side.

To eliminate some of the confusion with this asana, it is helpful to remember that whichever knee is in the air will be the guide for which arm is extended and the direction you will turn. For instance, if the left knee is in the air, then the left arm will be extended and you will be twisting to the left. This asana gives an unusual spiral twist to the entire spinal column. It also exercises the internal organs as well as limbering the hips and shoulders.

Fish—Lie on the back with the arms close to the body, palms down. Inhale, raising the chest off the floor, supporting yourself with the elbows.

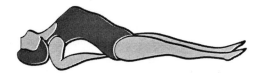

Arch your back and rest the top of your head on the floor, carefully walking (sliding) one elbow at a time toward the hips. Breathe deeply while holding the pose.

Expand the chest, lifting toward the ceiling. Lift the neck carefully, then slowly release the posture.

This strengthens the waist, spine and back muscles, helps asthma, massages the neck and shoulders and opens up the thyroid area.

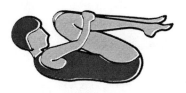

Knee Squeeze—Lying on the back, bring the knees to the chest. Wrap the arms around the knees, then slowly lift the head trying to touch the forehead to the knees. Try to relax the shoulders and have the feet flexed.

Have only one knee bent to the chest with the arms wrapped around the knee. The head and opposite leg are on the floor.

Inhale first, then, exhaling, raise the leg and head slowly off the floor until they form a "V," keeping that leg straight. Breathe shallowly as you hold

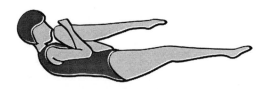

the posture. Inhale as you slowly lower the straightened leg and head to about one inch from the floor. Repeat the raising and lowering of the leg and head, then slowly let the leg and head go to the floor. Repeat with the opposite leg.

Now, with both legs flat on the floor, lift the head off the floor about one inch. Slowly turn the head from side to side three times. Stop in the center, and bring the head to the floor.

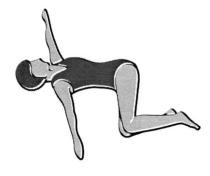

Side Rock—Lie flat on your back, your arms outstretched at shoulder level with the palms downward. Bring the knees up to the chest. Inhale, then exhaling, bring the knees to the right side of the body as you turn the head to the left. Breathe comfortably as you relax and hold the posture. Inhale as you bring the knees and head to the center of the body, then exhale as they go in opposite directions. Breathe comfortably as you hold the posture again, then return to the center and bring the legs down.

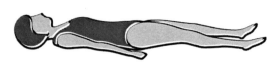

Savasana (Sponge, Corpse, or Relaxation Pose)—Lying flat on your back, place the feet about two feet apart. Put your arms a few inches from the sides with the palms up. Inch the shoulders down slightly, away from the ears. Tuck the chin forward slightly. Gently move all the different parts of the body to create a general condition of relaxation. Remind yourself to let the floor support you. Breathe slowly and deeply. Imagine yourself as being a passive observer, being aware of your body and mind, giving suggestions to yourself occasionally to relax.

Many of the yoga asanas concentrate on making the spine stronger and more flexible. This is an added benefit for those with epilepsy, since the spine is an important part of the central nervous system.

Meditation

A seizure may be a desperate signal from your central nervous system telling you that you need some rest. We each need to let the brain and nervous system idle in low gear for a few minutes each day. If you have epilepsy this quiet time is especially important because you may have a physical or chemical disorder which makes you more vulnerable to seizures when tension builds up.

The sensitivity from tension can be a burden on the nervous system. As you go through the day, talking to yourself and others, thinking, worrying, making decisions, experiencing all kinds of emotions, your brain wave activity is changing often from a fast pace to very slow intense activity. Even though the brain slows down often during your normal waking time, it isn't in a deep, relaxed state as in meditation.

There are many ways to get into a meditative state. Actually, there are as many different ways as there are human beings. No matter what technique is used, the common factor in all types of meditation is concentration, which leads to a state of detached non-thinking. Some of the most common types of meditation are:

Mantra—Concentrate on one word or syllable, such as "Om," "Love" or your own secret mantra.

Yantra—Create your own image or visualization.

Kasina—Meditate on an image (candle flame, etc.), closing the eyes occasionally, visualizing the image.

Chakras—Imagine energy (kundalini) coiling up to each chakra, which is a wheel of energy along the spine.

Tone or Tune—Concentrate on a musical tone or tune (short phrase).

Nasal Gaze—Close your eyes halfway, look inward to your nose.

Frontal Gaze—Looking toward your third eye in center of forehead, with eyes either closed or half-closed.

Steps for Meditation

A combination of repeating a mantra to yourself each time you exhale and frontal gaze is used in this example. If you prefer other methods of concentration, simply change step number 6 to suit your mood.

1. Sit up straight, shoulders down and relaxed, or lie in savasana (on your back, legs apart, arms at sides with palms up).
2. Be aware of your body, and send signals to any part which needs to relax. Tense, if necessary, then relax various parts of your body.
3. Be aware of your breathing. Breathe deeply and slowly. Count the breaths, i.e., 7 counts inhaling, 7 counts exhaling. After several rounds, forget about your breathing. Let it happen naturally.

4. If you have a problem or concern which is occupying your attention, visualize the problem, put the problem in an imaginary bubble in front of you. Let the bubble float upward and let it burst or float away. (Don't worry – you won't lose it. The problem will be there later if you want it back!)

5. Say to yourself, "I am going to relax and let myself meditate." Don't try to force yourself to meditate, and don't worry about whether you're doing it correctly or not. Simply go through the steps, and let it happen (passive volition). This phrase can be repeated whenever it is needed.

6. Start concentrating on your mantra (or whatever works for you). With your eyes closed, repeat the mantra to yourself each time you exhale. Occasionally look upward toward the center of your forehead for a few seconds. If other thoughts come to your mind, just notice them, look upward for a second, then go back to the point of concentration.

Very simply, meditation involves getting comfortable and relaxed, breathing deeply for a short time, focusing or concentrating, then letting go (doing "nothing").

Jacobson's Progressive Relaxation

This method works well for times when you need to direct your attention to certain parts of the body to become more relaxed. With Progressive Relaxation, you tense, then relax various parts of the body, part by part. This is based upon the very simple procedure of comparing tension against relaxation, much like yoga. Since you generally have very little awareness of the sensation of relaxation, you first tense a set of muscles as hard as you can until you feel real tension, even tenderness and pain in the muscles. Then you allow those muscles to relax, and try to become aware of, to feel internally, the difference between tension and relaxation.

Lie flat on your back, with your feet about two feet apart and your arms a few inches from your sides, palms up (yoga savasana pose). First think of the right leg. Slowly raise that leg off the floor. Hold it fully tensed. Point the toes, move the ankle. Concentrate on that leg, trying to keep the rest of the body relaxed. After a few seconds relax the muscles of that leg, letting it fall to the floor. Shake the leg gently from side to side, relax it fully, and forget about the existence of this leg. Repeat the same process with the left leg, then with each arm.

Next, bring the mind to the muscles of the pelvis, buttocks, anus and abdomen. Tense them, squeeze the buttocks together, then push the stomach muscles toward the floor. Now relax.

Move up to the chest and shoulder area. Raise the body up slightly, drawing the shoulder blades close together, stretching the chest upward. Hold for a few seconds, then let the chest area sink down, relaxed. Lift the head off the floor about one inch. Slowly turn the head from side to side three times, then stop at the center and let it down gently. Now turn the head from side to side while it is on the floor, then let it relax. Coming to the facial muscles, squeeze them all together, pouting, wrinkling the nose, squinting the eyes, gritting the teeth, making big chewing movements. Let the facial muscles relax.

Now that you have relaxed all the muscles of the body, allow your mind to go over the entire body, searching for any spots of tension. If you come across tension anywhere, mentally concentrate on this part and will it to relax. You can tense and relax any part again if it is needed.

This is complete relaxation. Even your mind is at rest now. You may keep watching your breath, which will be flowing in and out quite freely and calmly. Feel the cool, healing breath as you inhale, the warm breath taking away tension and negativity as you exhale. Watch the thoughts of your mind, without trying to take your mind anywhere. Feel as if you are the witness, not the body or the mind, but the true self or spirit.

After a few minutes, you may stretch, gently imagine that fresh energy is entering into each part of the body, then slowly sit up.

Autogenic Phrases

Saying phrases to yourself is another way to achieve relaxation. This can be combined with some of the other methods, done by itself, or changed to fit your individual needs. This was borrowed from hypnotic techniques, and is a combination of self-suggestion about relaxation and more advanced self-suggestion phrases for learning to control consciousness.

When doing this, you should either lie down flat on the floor or sit in a comfortable position. Do several rounds of deep breathing, then follow the following steps, saying the phrases to yourself slowly, pausing between each phrase as you let your body do what you're suggesting.

1. I feel very quiet.

2. I am beginning to feel quite relaxed.

3. My feet feel heavy and relaxed.

4. My ankles, my knees and my hips feel heavy, relaxed and comfortable.

5. My solar plexus, and the whole central portion of my body, feel relaxed and quiet.

6. My hands, my arms and my shoulders, feel heavy, relaxed and comfortable.

7. My neck, my jaws and my forehead feel relaxed. They feel comfortable and smooth.

8. My whole body feels quiet, heavy, comfortable and relaxed.

9. Continue visualizing and repeating any of the previous phrases silently for a minute, until you're ready to continue.

10. I am very relaxed.

11. My arms and hands are heavy and warm.

12. I feel very quiet.

13. My whole body is relaxed and my hands are warm, relaxed and warm.

14. My hands are warm.

15. Warmth is flowing into my hands, they are very warm.

16. I can feel the warmth flowing down my arms into my hands.

17. My hands are warm, relaxed and warm.

18. Continue visualizing and repeating any of the previous phrases silently for a minute, or until you're ready to continue.

19. My whole body feels quiet, comfortable and relaxed.

20. My mind is quiet.

21. I withdraw my thoughts from the surroundings and I feel serene and still.

22. My thoughts are turned inward and I am at ease.

23. Deep within my mind I can visualize and experience myself as relaxed, comfortable and still.

24. I am alert, but in an easy, quiet, inward-turned way.

25. My mind is calm and quiet.

26. I feel an inward quietness.

27. Continue using the phrases for a minute, allowing your attention to remain turned inward.

28. The relaxation and reverie is now concluded and the whole body is reactivated with a deep breath and the following phrases: "I feel life and energy flowing through my legs, hips, solar plexus, chest, arms and hands, neck and head. The energy makes me feel light and alive." Stretch.

Positive statements to yourself can also be very effective for relaxing at any time. Try to remember to stop many times each day. Take a few deep breaths, and say to yourself, "I am relaxed." Let your shoulders drop down, relaxed. Let your tongue lie in the bottom part of your mouth, the jaw relaxed. Even if you don't quite believe this as you're saying it, the subconscious mind will record the message and process it like data in a computer. You can also make statements concerning your well-being in general, such as, "I am very healthy," or "I enjoy life." Since the subconscious mind is like a recorder, the more times you repeat a positive statement, the more effective it will be. I will tell you more about positive thinking and how it can be helpful in a later chapter.

A General Guide To Keeping Yourself Relaxed

1. Stop many times each day, wherever you may be; breathe deeply. Let your shoulders and tongue drop, relax your jaw. Make positive statements to yourself.

2. Once or twice each day find a place to relax for 15 – 20 minutes. Practice some sort of relaxation. It can be one or any combination of the methods described in this chapter, which are: deep breathing, yoga asanas, meditation, progressive relaxation, autogenic phrases and positive thinking. Your way of relaxation might also be some other method or your own unique method. You can see the common thread with all these means of relaxing.

   a. Get yourself in a comfortable position.

   b. Breathe deeply for a minute or two.

   c. Tense or stretch then relax.

   d. Focus your thoughts on something simple.

   e. Forget everything else as much as possible.

   f. Feel connected to the entire universe or a Higher Power.

   g. Stretch, get up and enjoy the energy.

Sleep

Some people need more sleep than the average eight hours per night. Record in a journal the number of hours you sleep each night. Later, see if there is any correlation between seizures and how many hours you have slept the night before.

Lack of sleep makes you more vulnerable to seizures, so become aware of how much sleep you need to feel rested and alert. Stress management is especially important for days when you haven't had enough sleep and don't have time for a nap. Even five minutes of deep breathing while quieting the body and mind can be very helpful.

Chapter 5

Nutrition

Special Eating Habits Can Affect Epilepsy

"Our food must be our medicine—our medicine must be our food."
—Hippocrates

A well-balanced, nutritious diet is helpful in overcoming or preventing many illnesses and disorders, including epilepsy. Nutrition, like the other methods discussed in this book, is only one factor in health and disease. There are many unproven theories, hunches, fads and claims concerning the role of nutrition in health. What we eat, including supplements, can make a huge difference in our health. However, it is wise to take extraordinary claims of healing through vitamins, diets, etc., with a grain of salt. Since we are each unique, it is necessary to experiment, using suggestions and available information to find what works best for you.

I spent a lot of time experimenting, reading and learning, hoping to find a "miracle diet" to control my seizures, but also caring about optimum health in general. I achieved excellent general health before the epilepsy was conquered, so this was a rewarding fringe benefit. My efforts to learn about nutrition were confusing, since some "experts" suggested a high animal protein/low carbohydrate diet, while others said complete vegetarianism was the most nutritious diet, while others were positive that some variation in between these two extremes was the answer. Others claimed that mega-doses of certain vitamins and minerals was the answer.

An extreme diet which has been used mainly for children is the Ketogenic diet. This diet has been successful in reducing the severity of seizures for some children whose seizures couldn't be controlled in other ways. The Ketogenic diet gets its name because the high fat content of the diet results in conversion of fats-to-ketones that are utilized as an energy source in place of glucose (which are compiled of sugars). Carbohydrates must be severely restricted and all sugar must be eliminated for the diet to be effective. *Ketosis* (when there are elevated levels of ketones in the blood) usually occurs when people are fasting. A similar state can be induced by a very high fat diet. The child is hospitalized for several days when the diet is first started, with frequent visits afterward with the neurologist and dietitian. To be effective, the child must remain on the rigid diet. To find out more about this diet, talk with your neurologist and go to the recommended reading at the end of this book.

I discovered that fasting or skipping a meal would lower my seizure threshold (make me more likely to have a seizure). I would become weak and dizzy even when I didn't have a seizure. (By skipping a meal, I mean not eating at all.) I found that a nutritious snack such as some fruit, raw vegetables, cheese or nuts would give me the energy I needed.

Sugar, alcohol and caffeine were all to be avoided or taken in moderation if I wanted to be less vulnerable to seizures. Many people with epilepsy report these same observations about the relationship between their eating habits and seizures.

I was a vegetarian for several years, and I believe that made me more vulnerable to seizures. The brain and the nervous system need protein. It is very difficult for someone with epilepsy to get enough protein from other sources.

A high-protein diet with some similarities to the Ketogenic diet or the high-protein, high-fat diet recommended by Dr. Atkins, seems to be the logical solution. This would consist of:

- Protein: three small servings a day (nuts, eggs, cheese, milk, avocados, with meat at least once a day)
- Vegetables: 5 – 7 servings per day
- Fruit: 3 – 5 servings per day
- Little or no bread, cereal, potatoes
- Little or no sugar
- Little or no alcohol
- Little or no caffeine
- Plenty of water

If this diet seems too severe or impossible for you, modify it even more than this. Often the foods we crave the most are not those which are the most beneficial. We may crave a certain dessert with sugar or a delicious bread or some alcohol. This increases our blood sugar level or glucose, giving a temporary high, but then a rapid drop in blood sugar which could lead to low energy, depression, irritability and a possible seizure. We pay a high price for the instant gratification (short high)! The body will slowly make its own glucose from nutritious foods other than sugar, so sweeteners of any kind are not needed.

Don't overeat! Take small bites, chew food thoroughly. Roxanne Preble, EEG practitioner in San Francisco, suggests chewing each bite of meat 28 times. There will be a need to swallow liquid along with the chewing. Chewing sends a message to the brain, which sends a message to the stomach to prepare for digestion. As she tells her clients, "The stomach does not have teeth; it is designed to handle paste."

Do not skip meals. Research shows that overeating is one of the main causes of our ills, and that under-eating is the most important health and longevity factor. Russian statistics show that one common characteristic of all Russian centenarians is that they are all moderate eaters and have been such throughout their lives. Research has shown that overeating is the major cause of premature aging. Systematic under-eating (but not skipping meals), on the other hand, increases longevity, and decreases the incidence of the degenerative diseases. [1]

Drinking alcohol lowers the seizure threshold for many people with epilepsy. Some will tend to have a seizure the day after they have taken alcohol into their systems, while others will be more likely to have a seizure at the time they are drinking. Alcohol can interfere with the metabolism of anti-convulsant drugs. When combined with a high intake of alcohol, phenobarbitol and mysoline have both been associated with respiratory arrest (death because breathing just stops). For these reasons anyone wanting to be seizure-free would be wise to consume little or no alcohol.

Caffeine is a stimulant for the nervous system and will act in opposition to many anti-convulsant drugs. Since coffee and pop both contain caffeine (pop having harmful sweeteners as well), these must be avoided by people with epilepsy.

When you are in a social situation where others are drinking alcohol, coffee or pop, simply drink water, fruit or vegetable juice, herbal tea, or occasionally decaffeinated coffee. Some medication taken for the control of seizures causes stomach upset and the acid content of fruit juices could compound the problem, so omit fruit juices if you notice this problem for yourself.

A deficiency of B-6 (pyridoxine) can aggravate or cause seizures. Lack of B-6 will sometimes trigger a tic, twitch or tremor. It may cause tension, irritability, depression, insomnia, nervousness, severe halitosis, an inability to concentrate, lack of sex drive, edema (swelling, fluid retention) and dermatitis or eczema (red itchy skin).

Many women need extra B-6 while on oral contraceptives and before menstruation. The Pill so seriously depletes a woman of B-6 that infants born to her later may suffer from this deficiency.

Vitamin B-6 is essential for amino acid and fatty acid metabolism. But when large amounts of it are taken, the B-6 won't be absorbed by the body unless the other B vitamins (B complex and magnesium) are also increased.

Some foods rich in B-6 are: beef and chicken liver, lean muscle meats (white meat of chicken), fish, wheat germ, bananas, brewers yeast, brown rice, soybeans, whole grains, nuts and sunflower seeds.

Many drugs for epilepsy destroy folic acid, which is a member of the vitamin B complex, and must be taken with other B vitamins, especially B-12. Folic acid is usually included in a B complex supplement. The body does not easily absorb B-12. To make sure your body absorbs the B-12, use a sublingual tablet which dissolves under the tongue or a powder form which is dissolved in water first. You can buy boxes with packets of powdered vitamins. Look for those which have high amounts of all the B vitamins. The packets can be carried with you when you're away from home.

A deficiency of folic acid can cause anemia, diarrhea, hair loss, grayish-brown pigmentation, ulcers and menstrual disorders. It is absorbed much better when given in conjunction with vitamins C and E, as well as with vitamin B-12.

Good sources of folic acid are spinach, asparagus, liver, wheat bran, kale, endive, turnips, broccoli and potatoes. The RDA (recommended daily allowance) for folic acid is 400 mg. Extremely large amounts of folic acid may cause anti-convulsant drugs to lose their effectiveness, so it would be wise to check with a physician or nutritionist before taking folic acid in megadoses.

Manganese is sometimes at a low level in the blood of those with epilepsy. This trace mineral is essential for normal functioning of the nerve transmitter system. It also affects the way the body processes sugar and the function of the glandular system. Manganese is found in green leafy vegetables, whole grains, beans, peas, nuts, eggs and red meats.

A deficiency of the minerals calcium and magnesium can lower your seizure threshold. When taking supplements, calcium and magnesium must be taken at the same time if they are going to be beneficial. The most common ratio is two to one (twice as much calcium as magnesium); however, many experts suggest that the ratio be equal.

Calcium is vital to all body functions, especially in the proper utilization of other minerals as well as of vitamins D, A, and C. Calcium deficiency leads to hyper-excitability of the neuromuscular system resulting in irritability, nervousness, tingling and crawling sensations, muscle twitching, cramps, headache, premenstrual tension and menstrual cramps, periodontal problems, bleeding gums, insomnia and convulsions.

Magnesium is essential for vitamin C and sugar metabolism, and is involved in energy production. A deficiency of magnesium is characterized by mental confusion, delirium, jerky movements, convulsions, and hypersensitivity to light, noise and other stimuli.

When the "enrichment" of flour and bread was started, many millers began to add about three times as much calcium to bread as is lost in milling the flour, in order to make white bread and processed cereals. Some bakers add a large amount of calcium, but most don't add magnesium. This creates an imbalance, since calcium and magnesium are needed to help metabolize each other. Much of the manganese is also removed during the "enriching" process. The amount of "enrichment" is optional and the amount of vital nutrients removed from the flour and bread is seldom, if ever, replaced.

Calcium is supplied by milk, yogurt, buttermilk, green leafy vegetables, tofu, sunflower seeds, nuts and beans. Good sources of magnesium are cereals, especially buckwheat, and sesame seeds.

Some people with epilepsy are deficient in vitamin D. The best sources of vitamin D is from the sun. When the ultraviolet sunlight strikes the skin, the skin makes its own vitamin D. A few minutes in the sun will provide your daily dose of vitamin D. More is definitely not better!

Vitamin D is not found in many foods. Those that do contain it are oils of some fish, mostly halibut and cod. Egg yolk contains some and milk is "vitamin D-enriched."

A tremendous oversupply of vitamin D is dangerous. Like vitamin A, it is a fat-soluble vitamin whose excess is stored in the liver. The water-soluble vitamins' excess can be eliminated easily by the body. The U.S. recommended daily allowance (RDA) is 400 I.U. for vitamin D. Anti-convulsant drugs can lead to deficiencies of vitamin D and folic acid because they increase the turnover rate of these vitamins in the body. For this reason, people with epilepsy may need a higher intake of vitamin D than the RDA

Zinc is sometimes recommended for those with epilepsy to help keep the seizure threshold high. Zinc is an essential mineral that is involved with vitamin B-1 metabolism, protein metabolism and carbohydrate digestion. Good sources of zinc include liver, legumes, spinach, watercress and oysters.

Lecithin plays an important part in a healthy nervous system. Egg yolk, soybean oil and brain tissue are good sources of lecithin. Soy lecithin contains inositol, choline, chephaline and phosphorous. Phosphorous in the form of phosphoric acid forms a part of all bones and is present in large quantities in brain and nerve tissue.

For women whose seizures seem to be related to menstruation, a pre-menstrual vitamin complex is sometimes beneficial. These supplements commonly contain primrose oil, flaxseed oil, omega 3-6-9, which supply gamma linolenic acid (GLA), vitamin E, along with magnesium, vitamin B-6, vitamin B-12, calcium, magnesium and iron.

The amino acid, L-Tryptophan is one of the few substances capable of passing the blood-brain barrier. Tryptophan is no longer available over the counter in the U.S., but its synthetic version, 5-HTP, can be substituted.

Tryptophan has a variety of roles in mental activity. Serotonin, an inhibitory neurotransmitter in the brain, is dependent upon tryptophan for its formation. To have enough tryptophan you need enough B-6. Tryptophan is valuable in the treatment of sleep disorders, nervous disorders such as obsessive-compulsive behavior, depression and possibly seizure disorders.

L-Phenylalaline is also a neurotransmitter (a chemical that transmits signals between the nerve cells and the brain). It is turned into excitatory transmitters, norepinephrine and dopamine. This can be helpful for depression, memory and increased mental alertness.

The amino acid, L-Taurine, is found in very high concentration in excitable tissues such as the heart, skeletal muscles and the central nervous system. Taurine seems to be important in the development and function of the brain. Like tryptophan, it also acts as an inhibitory neurotransmitter. Studies at the University of Arizona[2] and in Canada[3] with rats have shown that taurine has a potent and long-lasting anti-convulsant action.

Taurine must be taken with L-Glutamine (glutamic acid). Glutamic acid has been shown to be important in sustaining mental ability, in the treatment of mental-emotional illness and alcoholism. While it is nutritionally non-essential for the body as a whole, it can be used in addition to glucose, as a fuel by brain cells. Low concentrations of taurine and glutamic acid are common for people with epilepsy.

You can experiment by taking one or two amino acids for a while, or you can simply take an amino acid complex containing all of them. You will get the most benefit from amino acids by taking them before or between meals.

Keep in mind that vitamins, minerals and all types of nutritional supplements are not medication, even though they often come in pill form. They are a source of concentrated food elements and should be taken in moderation. They are not meant to replace medicine or food.

Read articles, research reports and health food books to decide which foods and supplements might be beneficial to you. (Remember, everything that is written down is not necessarily proven or true.) When looking for information, some words to use as cues would be: brain, epilepsy, memory, concentration, seizures, mood, lethargy, and nervous system.

You probably won't completely change your eating habits in one day—in fact you may never completely change. However, you might try eliminating one harmful food at a time while substituting something both pleasant and nutritious. See if this has any effect on the number or intensity of your seizures, or just on your well-being.

If you like the results, continue with the substitution, then make another change, then another, etc. Naturally, there will be times when you will forget or ignore your new eating habits. Don't feel guilty or angry—it's not the end of the world. The stress caused by worrying about it could do more harm than the non-nutritious food. When those around you call you a "health food nut," ask them what's so nutty about wanting to be healthy!

----

[1] Paavo Airola, *Are You Confused?*, Phoeniz, AR: Health Plus: p. 52.

[2] Mantovani, et al, *Effects of Taurine on Seizures and Growth Hormone Release in Epileptic Patients,* Archives of Neurology XXXVI (1979): p. 672.

[3] R. Huxtable and H. Laird, *The Prolonged Action of Taurine on Genetically Determined Seizure-Susceptability,* Canadian Journal of Neurological Sciences V (1978) p. 220.

Chapter 6

Exercise For Helpful Energy On Your Journey

You could eat a wonderfully nutritious diet, practice biofeedback, yoga, meditation, and do a host of other healthful things for yourself, but without some vigorous aerobic exercise none of them would give you the optimum health you are looking for.

Our bodies need oxygen. We cannot go for more than five minutes without it. Many years ago, humans had to use their bodies a great deal. It was necessary to run, walk, and lift every day just to survive. Today, with cars, planes, boats and appliances we only use a small percentage of the physical power with which we are endowed. Inactivity increases our chances of developing arteriosclerosis and other types of heart disease, and leads to premature bodily aging. Exercise increases the metabolism, which helps to send blood, oxygen and essential nutrients to all part of the body, including the brain.

To make sure your brain and nervous system get this important energy, get some aerobic exercise—anything which will raise the heartbeat. Walking, jogging, running, hiking, bicycle riding, racquetball, tennis, swimming, dancing, martial arts, basketball, volleyball, jumping rope, and garden work are some good examples of this. Notice that many of these are outdoor activities. This is ideal, since you will be getting some of the invaluable vitamin D from the sun and some fresh oxygen while you are toning up your muscles.

If you don't drive, then walking or riding a bicycle can accomplish two things at once! You can travel to your destination while getting some healthful exercise. You will need to decide when it is safe to ride a bicycle. If you're still having a lot of seizures, you should wait until you're confident that you won't have a seizure while riding your bike.

A backpack will come in handy for the times when you need to carry groceries or other items. You might try going to the grocery store two or three times a week so you can fit everything into the backpack, or you might arrange for a ride to the store occasionally to pick up a large stock of staples.

For walking and jogging, you will need to increase your stamina gradually, first walking a short distance, then going further and faster as time goes on. Remember, jogging is not running rapidly; it is simply trotting lightly. This can be alternated with walking, especially at first. If it is possible, walk, hike or jog in the country or in a park, so you won't feel the pressure from sidewalks and streets.

Wear shoes that have good arch support and cushioned soles. Your legs can take you many places and will save you from at least some of the tiresome phone calls and requests for rides.

For days when the weather won't cooperate with some good outdoor aerobic exercise, keep a jump rope around or learn to use the hula hoop. You can raise your heartbeat and get some refreshing blood and oxygen all through your body in just a few minutes by jumping rope. If you prefer to use exercise equipment, join a gym or invest in an exercise machine. Be sure to try any equipment out first to see if it is something you will use regularly.

People who spend some time keeping fit usually show an increased ability to manage stress, have better eating habits, feel happier, and are more self-confident.

Some of the physiological benefits from exercise are a lowering of the cholesterol and fats in the blood, as well as decreased heart rate, blood pressure and stress levels. Physical activity usually reduces joint stiffness, which is a blessing for those suffering from arthritis. Exercise is very beneficial for the arteries, heart and lungs. Physical activity is essential for improving your digestion and metabolism, to tone up your muscles, to maintain efficient lymph nerve and blood circulation, to prevent osteoporosis, to assure the normal function of all organs and glands, and to supply enough oxygen to facilitate efficient cell and brain function.

If you are completely out of shape, have a coronary problem, or for any reason feel that strenuous exercise could be harmful to you, you may want to tell a physician your plan to get more exercise. Be sure to work into any fitness program gradually, being kind to yourself without pampering. Warm up slowly, gradually increasing your speed and intensity to protect your muscles. A few yoga asanas, as described earlier in this book, or other stretching, done after exercising will help to prevent sore muscles.

Choose the type or types of exercise that are the most fun for you. There is no need to compete, either with others or yourself. Of course the confidence and satisfaction which comes from winning a game or seeing yourself progress is great, but it is more important to simply have a good time while participating in the activity.

Exercise is great for overcoming boredom, depression and a lack of energy. It takes some willpower to get yourself going and to keep up with the exercise program. If you're having trouble getting started, simply walk around the block in the beginning, then increase your time gradually. The results will be well worth the effort!

Chapter 7

Music and Healing

"Music can be transcendent. For a few moments it makes us larger
than we really are, and the world more orderly than it really is. We
respond not just to the beauty of the sustained deep relations that are
revealed, but also to the fact of our perceiving them. As our brains are
thrown into overdrive, we feel our very existence expand and realize
that we can be more than we normally are, and that the world is more
than it seems. That is cause enough for ecstasy."

—*Robert Jourdain, Music, The Brain, and Ecstasy*

Music is wonderful for entertainment and enjoyment; it is also a vital
food that can nourish our minds and bodies. Great music, carefully
selected, can change our moods, energize us, calm us, improve our
mental focus, lift us up spiritually, and help us to become healthier.
Music has a direct effect on the EEG (brain wave activity). It can be
used as a stimulant, energizing and quickening brain activity, helping
us to focus and think more clearly, or it can help us to relax and ease
tension, equalizing the brain waves. Music can promote balance in
the personality. Music can prevent illness at the prephysical, energy-
imbalance level. Noise is the opposite of music. It is "sound gone crazy,"
failing to find any agreement or harmony with the universe, and can
be harmful.

Dr. Oliver Sacks, a neurologist who has written many papers and books
on neurology, and done studies on Parkinson's Disease, Tourette's
Syndrome, and Alzheimer's, has said, "Whenever I get a book on
neurology or psychology, the first thing I look up in the index is music,
and if it's not there, I close the book."

We are surrounded by music. The universe is a complete harmony of
many sounds—many lives interacting and vibrating together as they fill
the silence. All this energy can end up as harmony or as noisy discord.
The music we choose to listen to contributes to our energy. Music is the
positive pole of sound; it attunes us to powerful waves of life energy
and to the unfathomable source of all good.

The use of music has been shown to lower blood pressure, basal
metabolism and respiration rates. Music increases the production of

endorphins in the brain. Endorphins help to reduce pain, and salivary immunoglublin, which speeds healing, reduces infection, and controls heart rate. Music is often used in drug and alcohol detoxification and as an aid for those with learning disabilities. It has also been helpful with Alzheimer's patients, as well as the chronically or temporarily ill, the injured, and the dying.

Countless research studies have been done on the benefits of music for healing. In fact, there are over 900,000 references on music and healing. Following are some of these studies:

Studies by psychologist Janet Lapp at California State University, Fresno, have shown that migraine patients who started to and continue to listen regularly to their favorite music have one-sixth as many headaches as before.[1]

Dr. Raymond Bahr, head of the Coronary Care Unit at Baltimore's St. Agnes hospital says, "For adult patients, half an hour of music produces the same effect as ten milligrams of Valium." [2]

Premature babies at UCLA in Los Angeles and at Georgia Baptist Medical Center in Atlanta gained weight faster and used oxygen more efficiently; and babies at Tallahassee Memorial Regional Medical Center had shorter stays in the Intensive Care Unit when music was played for them daily, compared with babies in control groups without music.[3]

The cells of your body respond to music. There is practically no other human cultural activity which is so pervasive and which reaches into, shapes and often controls so much of human behavior with invisible vibrations. Since we cannot see the vibrations of sound, it is difficult to explain how that energy is capable of changing matter, including the electrical activity of the brain. This is Quantum Physics, and it is being used more and more with modern research.

The word "quantum" really means a very tiny, minute change. It is often misused as meaning "huge," such as a "quantum leap." A tiny (or quantum) change or bit of progress can have major effects on our awareness and health. Many ancient cultures (China, Middle East, India) have been investigating this phenomenon for thousands of years.

Sound can create physical forms and shapes that influence our health, consciousness and behavior. Ernst Chladni discovered that powdery particles scattered on a metal plate would respond to vibrations produced by running a cello bow across the edge of the plate. Different frequencies (high, low, etc.) would cause the particles to arrange themselves into complex, geometrically precise patterns. Each note produces an individual pattern that appears every time it is played; the frequency depends upon the size and thickness of the plate.

Deepak Chopra, author of *Quantum Healing,* says, "Where is the music? You can find it at many levels—in the vibrating strings, the trip of the hammers, the fingers striking the keys, the black marks on the paper, or the nerve impulses produced in the player's brain. But all of these are just codes; the reality of music is the shimmering, beautiful, invisible form that haunts our memories without ever being present in the physical world."

Of course, we process music by auditory function, with our ears, but also by body absorption. Sounds create messages to the brain that expand throughout the body. The body receives messages from the vibrations of the sounds, and sends messages to the brain. The body and mind cannot be separated. This will dramatically change the EEG, skin electromagnetic field, hormonal balance, and state of consciousness. The heartbeat and breathing both slow down or speed up along with changes in tempo and volume of the music. This synchronization is labeled "entrainment."

Each individual experiences a unique response to the same music. Musicians and non-musicians react differently, as do type A and type B personalities. We now know that music affects the EEG in the entire cortex, not, as once thought, just a part of the brain.

For scientific evaluation, EEG (brain waves) are divided into four major frequency "bands" or cycles per second, using Greek letters for naming them.

Beta: focused attention, concentration

Alpha: general relaxation, meditation

Theta: daydreaming, creativity, deep meditation

Delta: deep dreamless sleep

These brain waves are described in more detail in Chapter 3.

In a study by Ramos, Corsai and Cabrera, 1989, amateur musicians were exposed to silence, music, and infants crying, while measuring EEG response. All the subjects related the music as pleasant stimulation and the crying as unpleasant. Theta relative power was significantly higher while listening to music and lower during the crying. Beta power did not change, and there were no interhemispheric changes or correlations noted.

These results were just the opposite for non-musicians. All the subjects showed significant EEG changes across the board, not lateralized on either side of the brain nor localized. [4]

Other studies using professional musicians and non-musicians who listened to music have shown a difference in which side of the brain is activated the most. The professional musicians utilized more of the left side of the brain, and the non-musicians utilized more of the right side of the brain.

Regardless of the slight differences in the parts of the brain being activated, dancing, listening to and/or performing music activates more parts of the brain than any other activity. Nearly every cognitive part of the brain is involved in listening to music, and when we move to the music, as in dancing, many of the motor areas are involved as well.

Chanting or humming a continuous tone for several minutes has been shown to promote relaxation and healing. To chant along with a CD or to make up your own Gregorian chant-like sounds is like having a brain massage!

We know that music can contribute to healing. Now, which type of music is best? You can find lists of musical selections and types of music, with recommendations for helping specific illnesses or problems. There is research to prove that listening to Mozart's compositions raised IQ's and improved attention and behavior in children. Don Campbell has written several books on this subject, including "The Mozart Effect." Baroque classical music at a tempo of approximately 60 beats per minute has been shown to promote serenity. Deciding which style of music and which selections to listen to is a lot like choosing the correct diet for losing weight. We are each unique, and we often find certain foods to include or avoid, often by trial and error. It may also take some trial and error experiments to find the music that works best for you.

For meditation and relaxation, Baroque, slow classical music with clear beautiful harmonies or Gregorian chant will probably work the best.(Gregorian chant uses the natural rhythms of breathing.) To activate your brain and boost your attention level, high frequency sounds at a faster tempo will probably be more beneficial. However, music that is too loud and discordant may contribute to hearing loss as well as upsetting your energy field. Whenever you listen to or perform music, be aware of the profound effect the invisible energy is having on you.

What ultimately works in choosing the correct music is to select music that pleases you and helps you to achieve the mood and balance that you want.

Listening to background music can help create a dynamic balance between the more logical left and the more intuitive right hemispheres. Mozart, Baroque or any steady classical music can help to steady your conscious awareness and increase your mental organization. For "loosening up," listen to romantic, jazz or classical music from the Romantic period.

There are five basic variations in music which affect your state of being.

1. Tempo: the speed of the music; fast, moderate or slow.

2. Dynamics: the volume of the music; loud or soft.

3. Pitch: the frequency of the music; high or low.

4. Timbre: the tone of the particular instrument or voice.

5. Style: Classical, Romantic, Jazz, Celtic, etc.

For best results, don't listen to music for more than three hours at a time. If you find that you've had music on for three hours, turn it off and take a break from the music.

Following are some general guidelines for choosing music:

Meditation and Non-thinking: Gregorian Chant, which uses the rhythms of natural breathing, creates a sense of relaxed spaciousness and relaxation. Humming or Toning can create a feeling of oneness with the universe. New Age or improvised music with no dominant rhythm or predictable harmony can induce a state of relaxed attention.

Study or Work: Slower Baroque music (Bach, Handel, Vivaldi, Corelli) creates a mentally stimulating environment for study or work, while imparting a sense of order and stability.

Concentration, Memory and Spatial Perception: Classical music (Haydn and Mozart) has clarity and elegance. The EEG (electroencephalograph or brain waves) of a person with epilepsy (also ADD and ADHD) commonly produces high amplitude bursts of theta. Neurologists often use the EEG to diagnose epilepsy by spike and wave activity, which is high bursts of theta (slower brain wave activity) alternated with bursts of beta (faster brain wave activity). Music played at a moderate or moderately fast tempo, without too many abrupt changes in dynamics (loud and soft) helps to normalize the EEG. In Concertos, Sonatas and Symphonies, look for tempo markings or sections titled, "Andante, Allegretto, or Allegro."

Compassion, Love, Emotions: Romantic music (Schubert, Schumann, Tchaikovsky, Chopin, Liszt) emphasizes expression and feeling.

Creativity, Daydreaming: Impressionist music (Debussy, Fauré and Ravel) is based on free-flowing musical moods, and evokes dreamlike images. It can put you in touch with your unconscious.

Inspiration, Uplifting: Jazz, the Blues, Dixieland, Soul, Gospel, Calypso and other dance forms can release deep joy and sadness, and affirm our common humanity.

Awaken and Energize: Salsa, Rhumba, Maranga, Macarena, and other South American music have a lively rhythm and beat that can get the whole body moving. Samba has the rare ability to soothe and awaken at the same time.

Well-being: Big band, Pop, Top-40 and Country can inspire light to moderate movement, engage the emotions, and create a sense of well-being.

Stimulation: Fast, loud Classical music or Rock music can stir the passions, stimulate active movement, mask pain and release tension. Rock music can also create tension, discord and pain if it is too loud or dissonant, or when we are not in the mood to be energetically entertained.

When you want to relax, meditate, go to sleep or slow down in any way, start with music at a moderate or faster tempo to match your metabolism, then gradually switch to slower and slower music. When you want to wake up or have more energy, start with slow, quiet music, then gradually switch over to louder pieces with a faster tempo.

Remember how it feels when you hear a piece of music you love when you had forgotten about it? There are favorites of yours and those labeled "everyone's favorites." They are favorites because they have a special vibration, harmony, rhythm, melody, etc., which can't be analyzed or explained.

You are unique. Experiment with different types of music, and be aware of the effects each style of music has upon your mental, emotional and physical well-being. Choose music that appeals to you. This will change, sometimes very quickly, within a few minutes or hours, depending upon your mood. Listen to yourself. You are the ultimate guide and healer.

----

1. *Reader's Digest,* 141.174 – 178. Aug. 1992.

2. *Parents Magazine,* 62.14. 1999.

3. *Harp Therapy Journal,* 1999.

4. *Body, Mind, and Music,* p. 101, 1998, Laurie Riley.

Chapter 8

Medication: Some Facts About The Side Effects

It is wonderful that we have the scientific knowledge to create all the helpful medicine available to us today. Any medication can have good effects (help to control seizures) along with bad (side) effects. It helps your physician if you are an informed patient.

Research is continually being done to find which drugs are effective for which types of epilepsy and which are effective for each individual. For those people who are believed to have more than one type of epilepsy, more than one medicine may be taken, making the treatment more complicated. Dosages vary, depending upon the degree of absorption and the rate of metabolism of the medication (how quickly it gets into the system). This is known as your blood level, and should be checked at a medical lab occasionally.

Other medications may decrease the effectiveness of anticonvulsant drugs, so a physician needs to know if you are taking any other medication not related to epilepsy. Even common drugs such as aspirin, caffeine and alcohol can have an effect on anticonvulsant drugs. Drugs that stimulate ("uppers" in street language) the nervous system can lower the seizure threshold, thereby making it easier for seizures to occur. Stimulants include cocaine, Ritalin, amphetamines and caffeine. Drugs that sedate can also lower the seizure threshold. Some drugs which sedate are marijuana, alcohol and tranquilizers. Drugs at either end of the spectrum should be avoided.

Doctors sometimes advise their patients with epilepsy not to use birth control pills. Oral contraceptives contain the hormones estrogen and progesterone, and researchers suspect hormones may play some part in epilepsy. Water retention may influence the development of seizures, and in some women oral contraceptives cause the body to hold more water than usual.

Many people experience stomach upset from taking anticonvulsant medication. Here are some basic rules you can follow which will help to prevent stomach upset.

1. Don't take the morning dose with just a cup of coffee.

2. Take your morning dose with water, then eat something. By doing this, you have diluted the medication in your stomach, thereby reducing your chances of stomach upset. With the exception of Tegretol, most drugs absorb faster and in greater quantities if they are taken before a meal.

3. Tegretol is better absorbed if taken on a full stomach. You will have less stomach upset (and fewer side effects like dizziness, lack of coordination, blurred vision, etc.) from this drug if you take the dose right after a meal (on a full stomach).

4. Some people who take Depakene report less or no stomach upset from the drug if they avoid acidic foods such as orange juice, grapefruit juice and coffee while Depakene is in the stomach. Depakote, which is less irritating to the stomach, is sometimes substituted for Depakene.

There are a few things which apply to any of the anticonvulsant medicines. First, the use of any anticonvulsant drug may cause personality changes, confusion, drowsiness and other side effects.

Next, it would be wise to check with a physician if you are pregnant, since there is some association between the use of anticonvulsant drugs by women with epilepsy and an elevated incidence of birth defects in children born to these women. Of course, the effects of seizures on the unborn fetus could cause as much damage as the medicine, so you will need to do some careful planning with your physician if you are pregnant or are planning to be.

Always start a medication slowly and gradually, keeping a record of the number of seizures and watching for any side effects. Withdrawal or substitution should also be done very gradually and under the supervision of your physician, since abrupt withdrawal may precipitate status epilepticus, a life-threatening situation.

Following are the benefits and side effects of some of most commonly used medications for epilepsy. The list of side effects may seem long and frightening. Keep in mind that you may experience none or only a few mild side effects.

Celontin

Used mostly for petit mal (absence) seizures.

Possible Side Effects:

* Nausea, vomiting, anorexia (loss of appetite), diarrhea, weight loss, abdominal pain, and constipation.

* Drowsiness, inability to coordinate voluntary muscle movements, dizziness, irritability and nervousness, skin rash, headache, blurred vision, fear of light, hiccups, and insomnia.

* Confusion, instability, mental slowness, depression, hypochondriacal behavior (imagined illness) and aggressiveness.

* May increase the frequency of grand mal (tonic clonic) seizures in some patients.

Clonopin

Used mostly for absence (petit mal) seizures and decreasing the frequency, amplitude, duration and spread of discharge in minor motor seizures.

Possible Side Effects:

* Central nervous system depression, drowsiness, inability to coordinate voluntary muscle movements, behavior problems, confusion, depression, suicide attempts, forgetfulness, slurred speech, headache, hallucinations, hysteria, increased libido (sexual desire), insomnia and psychosis.

* Chest congestion, runny nose, shortness of breath, hypersecretion in respiratory passages, rapid heartbeat, hair loss, edema (swelling of tissue).

* Anorexia (loss of appetite), weight loss or gain, urinary infection, muscle weakness, pains.

* May increase or precipitate the onset of grand mal (tonic clonic) seizures.

Clobazam (Frisium)

Adjunctive therapy in broad range of seizures, including myoclonic infantile spasms and petit mal (absence) seizures.

Possible Side Effects:

* Sedation, tiredness, muscle weakness, drowsiness, unsteadiness, irritability, weight gain/loss.

Clonazepam (Rivotril)

Adjunctive therapy with atonic, myoclonic, infantile spasms and petit mal (absence) seizures.

Possible Side Effects:

* Lethargy, dizziness, nausea/vomiting, increase in bronchial secretions, weight loss/gain, slurred speech.

Depakene (Sodium Valproate)

For the control of simple and complex absence (petit mal), tonic clonic idiopathic and partial complex seizures. Also used in adjunctive therapy where there are multiple seizure types. Chemically unrelated to other drugs used to treat seizure disorders.

Possible Side Effects:

* Nausea, vomiting and indigestion, diarrhea, abdominal cramps and constipation.

* Both anorexia (loss of appetite) with some weight loss and increased appetite with weight gain have been reported.

* Drowsiness, emotional upset, depression, psychosis, aggression, hyperactivity and behavioral deterioration. Hair loss, skin rash, weakness, irregular menstrual periods.

* Over-dosage may result in deep coma.

Dilantin (Phenytoin)

Used to control grand mal (tonic clonic) and psychomotor (complex partial) seizures.

Possible Side Effects:

*   Liver toxicity, reversible lymph node enlargement, low white blood cell count, skin rash, nystagmus (a swinging, vibration of the eyes, especially when looking to the side), ataxia (inability to coordinate voluntary muscular movements), slurred speech, mental confusion, drowsiness, dizziness, insomnia, transient (changing quickly) nervousness, motor twitchings, headache, nausea, vomiting and constipation, affects birth control pill, gum overgrowth.

*   May make petit mal (absence) seizures worse.

Mysoline (Primidone)

For the control of grand mal (tonic clonic), psychomotor (complex partial) and focal epileptic seizures.

Possible Side Effects:

*   Ataxia (inability to coordinate voluntary muscle movements) and vertigo (dizziness).

*   Drowsiness, appetite loss, irritability, nausea, hyperactivity, mood or personality changes, depression.

Phenobarbital

A long-acting barbiturate acting as a central nervous system depressant for use as a sedative or anticonvulsant with Dilantin.

Possible Side Effects:

*   Central nervous system depression, drowsiness, lethargy, insomnia, slurred speech, mental confusion and vertigo (dizziness).

*   Emotional disturbances and phobias may be accentuated.

*   Transient nervousness, motor twitchings, headache, nausea, vomiting, hyperactivity, mood changes, depression, behavioral/ learning problems.
*   Allergic reactions including swelling, particularly of the eyelids, cheeks or lips.
*   Prolonged, uninterrupted use may result in psychic and physical dependence.

Tegretol (Carbamazepine)

For the control of partial seizures (psychomotor, temporal lobe), generalized tonic clonic seizures (grand mal), mixed seizure patterns which include the above, or other partial or generalized seizures.

Possible Side Effects:

*   Aplastic anemia, change in liver function, low white blood cell count, depression with agitation, dizziness, drowsiness, disturbances of coordination, confusion, headache, fatigue, blurred vision, visual hallucinations, speech disturbances, abnormal involuntary movements, talkativeness, skin rashes, impotence, nausea, vomiting, gastric distress and abdominal pain, renal (kidney) dysfunction, diarrhea, constipation, urinary frequency or retention, loss of appetite, dryness of the mouth.

*   Congestive heart failure, aggravation of hypertension (high blood pressure), hypotension (low blood pressure), edema (swelling of tissues), coronary artery disease.

*   Sometimes aching joints and muscles, as well as leg cramps.

Zarontin (Ethosuximide or Succinimide)

Used for petit mal (absence) seizures.

Possible Side Effects:

* Gastrointestinal symptoms occur frequently and include anorexia (loss of appetite), vague gastric (stomach) upset, nausea and vomiting, cramps, abdominal pain, weight loss and diarrhea.

* Drowsiness, hyperactivity, headache, dizziness, euphoria (an extreme sense of well-being), hiccups, irritability and ataxia (inability to coordinate voluntary muscular movements).

* Disturbance of sleep, night terrors, inability to concentrate, aggressiveness.

I have mentioned some of the most commonly used medications for epilepsy. If you want to find out more about any of them or about one which I didn't describe, look in *The Essential Guide to Prescription Drugs* by James W. Long, MD, or go to a library and ask for the *Physicians' Desk Reference (PDR)*. Check in the front of the PDR under "Product Name Index" to find the name of the medicine you're interested in, then turn to the pages where it is described.

Your pharmacist can also give you information about medications. Ask for the package insert for each bottle of medicine that the pharmacist receives from the drug company, giving all the pertinent clinical data about the contents.

You will likely never experience all of the side effects which are possible from the medicine you're taking, maybe none of them, so don't panic. However, it is good to be aware of the side effects so that if you do experience undesirable results you will know the cause. Sometimes all the side effects of a drug are not discovered during the initial testing, so tell your prescribing physician when you do notice undesirable side effects. It sometimes takes many reports from patients to impress on the scientific community that unknown side effects actually do exist. If the side effects are too irritating, you may want to talk with your physician about trying a different medication or about very carefully and gradually cutting back on the amount you're taking.

Of course, seizure control is a good effect (the desired effect) of anticonvulsant drugs when they work for you. You may decide that tolerating some bad side effects is a small price to pay for seizure control.

Try to work in cooperation with your physician concerning your medication, asking questions and listening, communicating your needs and feelings.

Keep in mind that I am NOT recommending self-treatment. I am providing information to help you become more knowledgeable. Do not make changes in your medication without consulting your attending physician.

Chapter 9

Self-Esteem

Epilepsy has a profound effect on self-esteem. If you have epilepsy, this "profound" statement is probably no great revelation.

One person who has seizures says, "Loss of control is one of the scariest things about epilepsy. For instance, the other day as I was coming out of a shop, I felt a little strange. The next thing I knew I was several blocks away, not knowing how I had gotten there."

Another person says, "My son won't admit to anyone that he has epilepsy because he thinks anyone who knows looks down on him or makes fun of him."

Yet another person adds in a cynical tone, "Sure, there's no discrimination against hiring or firing someone with epilepsy! They always find a way to get around it legally."

Feelings of helplessness, hopelessness, fear, anger, frustration, embarrassment and self-pity often accompany epilepsy. It is helpful to bring these feelings out in the open and talk about them. Learning better communication skills, assertiveness, self-exploration and affirmations are ways to increase self-esteem.

The best way to improve communication is by practice. If you don't drive and/or feel shy in social situations, you may have to put forth extra effort to find people with whom you can communicate. A support group can be an excellent way to become acquainted and share with others who have some of the same feelings and challenges as you do. You can find epilepsy support groups and organizations in your area by searching for Epilepsy Support Group on your favorite search engine, or check out some of the informational Websites listed in the back of this book.

Pursuing hobbies can be another excellent way to meet people and practice communication. Spending time at an activity which you enjoy and/or are good at is another way to build your self confidence, which will make communicating more pleasurable.

Listening is an important part of communication, and this is often disregarded. When another person is talking, try not to be thinking of what you're going to say next. Simply be there, listening. If you are interested in what the other person is saying, you may find yourself asking questions. Remind yourself that asking questions is not a sign of stupidity, and that you will not usually be laughed at for asking questions. On the contrary, the person who inquires often ends up more knowledgeable about life than those who are afraid to do so. Everyone appreciates having someone who will listen. Psychologists, psychiatrists, barbers, hair stylists, teachers, and ministers certainly understand that! A genuine interest and concern for others often prompts questions while taking away self-consciousness.

When you are doing the talking, express your feelings and thoughts as honestly as you can. Remind yourself that if you say something which you regret you can admit your blunder, apologize to yourself and/or the other person, then go on.

Assertiveness makes you feel better about yourself because you are honestly and courageously communicating what you feel, think and want—without putting someone else down.

Two other less desirable ways for communicating are aggressiveness and passivity. Avoid communicating your feelings, thoughts and needs aggressively by humiliating, dominating, controlling or attacking another person, often in anger.

It is also not desirable to use passive behavior by not standing up for your rights, or by agreeing with almost everything someone else says because you don't want any pressure or discomfort. There is often anger with passive behavior, but it is hidden or repressed.

Two key words when speaking assertively are, "I," and "No." Use sentences which begin with, "I," such as, "I feel _____,"
"I need _____," "I like _____,"
"I dislike _____," etc.

"No." can be one sentence. It isn't always necessary to explain, qualify or back down. You may have to repeat the sentence ("No.") many times to persistent people!

Self-exploration can be educational, painful, frightening, tiring and rewarding. Self-exploration often leads to change, and change is often accompanied by pain and fear. The increase in self-esteem after self-exploration and change makes the discomfort seem worthwhile. One method of self-exploration is to talk with a therapist (psychologist, psychiatrist, counselor, social worker, minister or friend), trying to clarify your needs, feelings, thoughts and desires. A support group can also be very helpful.

Another method of self-exploration is meditation, listening to your inner-self in a passive way. A problem or question can be answered during meditation by asking a question as you begin to meditate, then reminding yourself to forget about the question as you meditate. Even though the answer doesn't always come immediately in a direct way, much insight can be gained by this type of "quiet mind" searching.

The same thing can be accomplished while you're dreaming. As an example, before meditating or going to sleep, say to yourself, "I am going to learn what to do about _____."

Journal writing is still another technique for self-exploration. The writing doesn't have to be lengthy to be helpful. Learning about yourself from your writing may be postponed until you've been keeping a journal for some time. As you read over past writings, you may discover some patterns of thinking or behavior of any kind, and begin writing. This book was created as a result of my journal writing.

Making positive statements to yourself (affirmations) can be a valuable method for increasing your self-esteem, confidence and well being. Any or all of the things described in this book can contribute to your well being, and if you believe in yourself the results will be quicker and more lasting.

We have a tendency to talk to ourselves constantly, as you're probably very much aware if you have tried to meditate or quiet your mind. The subconscious mind records all this "chatter" and uses it as it thinks it's meant to be used. The subconscious cannot discriminate between negative and positive information. For this reason it is important to notice what you are saying, which many times is a common phrase that you don't even mean. If you have epilepsy, notice your repetitive sayings. See if you use the expression, "I about had a fit," or "I could have fainted," or "I about passed out," or "I can't stand any more of that."

Even if someone else says, "She just threw a fit!" your subconscious hears those phrases, and if repeated enough times, may act on them. When you are conscious of yourself or someone else using a phrase like this, say to yourself, "I won't really have a fit or seizure. I'm only surprised." (or angry, shocked, frustrated, etc.) Or simply say, "Cancel."

An affirmation you might use is, "I am free of seizures now." or "My brain cells are working in perfect harmony." Say the affirmation each day and say it aloud when you can. The brain is most open to suggestions when it is producing very slow brain waves, such as right after meditation, just before falling asleep or right after awakening. Repeat the phrase any time during the day when you happen to think of it, no matter how you think your brain may be operating.

If you want a statement about your general well-being, try the phrase given to people by the physician Dr. Emile Coue. In the beginning of the 20th century he cured thousands of people of every conceivable illness by having them repeat 20 times twice daily this affirmation to themselves:

"Every day in every way, I am getting better, and better and better!" Another general affirmation is, "I am a healthy worthwhile person."

Repeat any combination of statements which sound like they fit your needs, or create your own. A good rule is to begin with, "I am," add a few words, and end with the word, "now."

Affirmations should be positive and in the present tense. If you believe the statements you will see results very quickly. Even if you don't quite believe what you're saying to yourself, the statements will have an effect. It's not unusual to be skeptical at first; but if the affirmations are repeated enough times, your subconscious mind will finally start reacting to them.

Besides making affirmations, you can also visualize yourself in a healthful state. This, like affirmations, will have more power when you're in a very relaxed state. First, say to yourself, "My brain cells and nervous system are working well. Any defects are being healed naturally." Now, visualize what you think your brain looks like. The eyes should be closed. Imagine the brain perfectly in balance, everything flowing smoothly. Visualize the spinal cord, perfectly centered, with a stream of white energy radiating to and from the brain. Don't worry if you don't know exactly what your brain looks like. Just imagine each cell as being perfectly formed, everything in balance, functioning well. Keep repeating positive statements about your brain cells at the same time. The visualizing can be used for healing any part of yourself (and others) by concentrating on areas that need special attention.

You have seen, heard, or read about miraculous healings performed by healers who use such unconventional techniques as the laying on of hands, holy waters, psychic surgery or prayer. The implication is always that the healer possesses great healing powers.

The healing power is within ourselves; the healer only helps to release it. You do not need to know any special ritual or formula to accomplish the same things independently. It may seem easier to get started if you have some sort of pattern to go by, but you can create your own.

The following is a basic procedure to try when you want to be conscious of the powerful healing energy available.

If you meditate, the ideal time for this would be right after meditation. Get yourself comfortable and relaxed. Take several slow deep breaths, get yourself in a comfortable position, then proceed.

Say to yourself, "I am open to healing energy. It is radiating and cleansing, giving power to every part of my brain. More of the energy is flowing to any part of my body which needs an extra boost to heal itself."

Some people visualize the healing energy as green light, perhaps symbolizing growth. Others see it as golden light, symbolizing the sun. Some see it as white light. You may see it differently, since you are unique.

Enjoy the energy, give it a little direction, and notice the effects. This can be done as often as you want because you will never run out of this energy. It can be directed to others, either near or far away, by visualizing the energy going from your body, through your arms, out your fingers, to the person who needs to be healed.

You share this energy often when you touch others; it is sometimes called love, empathy or compassion. This energy is stronger when you are aware of it and give it some direction.

Since you are unique you may need to alter some of the methods I describe, or create some of your own. Keep in mind that you can get suggestions, orders, prescriptions, drugs, etc., from others, but it is how you act upon all of this which will be important.

Examine yourself when you immediately scoff at any statement to the effect that, "Epilepsy can be overcome," and "You can be responsible for your life and health." Perhaps you are afraid that you might not master it, and you would then feel embarrassed, discouraged or that you're a failure. Maybe the epilepsy removes you from some stressful situation.

Ask yourself, "Are there any benefits from my seizures?"

Sometimes feelings like these don't show up until you've started to gain control over your seizures. If this happens, be aware of yourself. Use positive statements for this, too, such as, "I am well, strong, and in control of my life. I don't really need to black out and have a seizure for any reason." Talk with someone at times like these if you feel the need.

Just because you hit a roadblock in the journey (and you could have many), don't be discouraged and give up! It is common to have setbacks as you progress. When you do have a seizure, even if the probable cause was your lack of self-discipline, forgive yourself. Remind yourself to learn what you can from the experience, and go on.

The following quotation describes how your state of mind can have a powerful impact on your health.

"Healing is accomplished the instant the sufferer no longer sees any value in pain. Who would choose suffering unless he thought it brought him something, and something of value to him? He must think it is a small price to pay for something of greater worth. For sickness is an election; a decision."[1]

Illness is not something you imagine or dream up, nor should you feel guilt or shame if you have an illness or disorder. There is no human being who has never been ill. Many of us with epilepsy know that it is often the result of a physical event, such as brain damage at birth, or from an accident or infection.

How we react and what we do to overcome or live with the epilepsy is what is important. We could complain, worry, feel sorry for ourselves, be relieved of responsibility, use seizures as an escape and get lots of sympathy all the rest of our lives. On the other hand, we could say, "I have epilepsy for some reason. I am going to try to find out why. I am going to use this to my advantage to learn more about life. I am going to read, write letters, make phone calls, experiment, ask questions, listen, contemplate, talk with others who have epilepsy, and use everything within my power to find out how I can have more control over seizures."

You may find many people around you who are very skeptical of the power of the mind. Many will be sure that epilepsy is a disorder which is completely uncontrollable. It doesn't matter why they think this.

Whatever their reasons, you need to learn to tell them politely that you do not agree with their views, and that you are going to control your seizures as well as possible, going to feel in balance, and going to enjoy most of your life.

This could mean learning to live with seizures, controlling some seizures, or becoming free of seizures. You won't be able to convince everyone of your positive views and shouldn't waste your time trying. If someone is interested and wants to hear what you're doing, of course share with them, but remember not to be discouraged by others' negative comments and attitudes.

Informed, understanding loved ones and friends who are optimistic can be an important source of strength. If those who are close to you are skeptical, the best way to prove your point will be by example. This will take patience since it may take a long time, and they could see you stumble and fall (have seizures) many times on your journey.

If you have epilepsy, do not let yourself feel unworthy because of it. There have been all kinds of people with this problem. It is believed that many unusually bright or gifted people had epilepsy.

Included are the musical geniuses, Handel, Berlioz, Mendelssohn, Mozart, Tchaikovsky and Paganini; religious leaders, Buddha, Mohammed and St. Paul; famous statesmen and rulers, Alexander the Great, Julius Caesar, Alfred the Great and William Pitt; writers Byron, de Maupassant, Dostoevski, Edward Lear, Charles Dickens, Dante and Socrates; among the artists are Van Gogh, famous in modern art, and Leonardo Da Vinci, who gave the world "Mona Lisa" and "The Last supper." Alfred Nobel, remembered each year when the prize winners are announced was an engineer, inventor, writer, manufacturer, industrialist and humanitarian who had seizures all his life.

Imagine your job of becoming as seizure-free as possible as being like climbing a ladder. You climb toward your ultimate goal, a step at a time, even if you can't see the very top of the ladder. Each step on the ladder is a short-term goal that you reach for. A typical goal might be stopping your first seizure, or when you haven't had any seizures for one day, or one week, or one month, or one year.

When you reach each goal, you can celebrate, congratulate yourself, then set a new one to strive for (go one more step up the ladder). At times when you're discouraged and tired, don't stop! Think how you would feel if you found that you only had one more step to go when you tossed everything in and gave up!

As Thoreau wrote, "If you have built castles in the air, your work need not be lost; that is where they should be. Now put the foundations under them."

----

1. © 1975, *Foundations for Inner Peace, A Course in Miracles, Manual for Teachers,* p.16, used by permission.

Ten Steps to Controlling Your Epilepsy

These ten steps can really help you or a loved one control seizures and take back control of life. But it's up to you to take the steps or encourage your loved one to take them.

1. **Consult with a Qualified Doctor**
   Seek the advice of a competent doctor (MD, DO, or neurologist) with whom you feel you can communicate easily. Ask questions. Report seizures, side effects of medication, and any information you think could be linked to your problem. To help your doctor help you as much as possible, you'll want to start tracking your seizures, their times, what you ate beforehand, what your physical and mental states were at the time and anything else that may have had to do with your seizure.

2. **Search Out Information**
   Learn everything you can about epilepsy and your general health. Read, ask questions and search the Internet for facts. Investigate alternative and complementary methods of healing, such as biofeedback, music therapy, acupuncture, acupressure, homeopathic medicine and chiropractic treatment. Get to know others who have epilepsy through a support group.

3. **Neurofeedback (EEG Biofeedback)**
   Train with a competent therapist as you learn to inhibit undesirable slow spike-and-wave brain wave patterns and to produce safe, healthy electrical activity within your brain.

4. **Stress Management**
   Experiment with and learn stress reduction methods, such as deep breathing, meditation, hand temperature biofeedback, yoga, autogenic phrases or progressive relaxation. Persistently practice at least two of these methods until it becomes easy, almost automatic, for you to achieve a state of relaxation. Set aside 20 minutes each day to let yourself unwind.

5. **Positive Thinking and Vibrational Energy**

   Believe in yourself and your natural healing energy. Twenty times twice each day repeat a positive present-tense affirmation to yourself. Some examples are: "My brain, central nervous system and body are healthy." "I feel vibrant, balanced and healthy." "I am free of seizures." Visualize each brain cell or your entire brain as being in perfect working order, balanced, in harmony, functioning smoothly. Be persistent with your affirmations and visualizations. Each thought changes your entire metabolism and the vibrational energy around you. Be aware of your thoughts.

6. **Nutrition**

   Eat a healthful diet, being sure to get plenty of vegetables, protein and fruit. Eliminate or cut back on sugar, carbohydrates, salt, alcohol and caffeine. Don't skip meals. Read about and experiment with supplements, such as: multi-vitamin/mineral complex, B complex (especially B-6, B-12 and folic acid), lecithin, amino acids and calcium/magnesium.

7. **Exercise**

   Supply your cells and brain with enough oxygen by getting some aerobic exercise (anything which will raise the heartbeat) at least three times per week. Walking, hiking, jogging, running, bicycle riding, tennis, dancing swimming, basketball, volleyball, jumping rope or garden work are good examples.

8. **Adequate Sleep**

   Observe your sleeping habits; find out how many hours of sleep you need each night. Lack of sleep makes many people more vulnerable to seizures (lowers the seizure threshold). On days when your previous night's sleep hasn't been adequate, take a nap if possible, practice some type of stress reduction and be sure to eat a nutritious diet, not skipping any meals.

9. **Self Awareness**

    Keep a journal. Become more aware of your feelings of fear, anger, hopelessness, worthlessness, as well as your hopes, fantasies, dreams and needs. Learn better ways of coping with the undesirable feelings and to forgive yourself for not being perfect. Find ways of fulfilling your needs, desires and hope. Talk to friends and loved ones. Seek counseling when you feel that you need professional help as you get to know yourself better.

10. **Self Esteem**

    Search within yourself, admit and accept your positive attributes, many of which are unique. Forgive yourself for mistakes and imperfections. Make a list of your past accomplishments and attributes, perhaps asking a loved one or friend to assist you. Be open to suggestions and praise from others, to inspirations and to your creativity as you grow to more fully appreciate yourself.

Final Word

It has been my intention to give you ideas, inspiration and hope. Now it's up to you to try any or all of these suggestions. Please let me know what has helped you from this book, as well as other solutions and ideas. Maybe the next edition will have another chapter with your success story!

Appendix 1: Things that Lower the Seizure Threshold

Here is a list of some of the things that can lower the seizure threshold level or act as seizure precipitants:

- Emotional stress, such as: divorce, death of someone close, anxiety, embarrassment or fear, feeling bad about oneself (80 – 90% of seizures are caused by stress.)

- Excitement

- Boredom, lack of activity or interest

- Extreme fatigue

- Lack of adequate, regular sleep

- Poor nutrition (eating junk food or skipping meals)

- Hypoglycemia (low blood sugar)

- Consumption of alcohol

- Heat and/or humidity

- Consumption of large amounts of food or drink at one time

- Allergies

- Menstrual cycle

- Bladder too full (putting off urination)

- Constipation

- Fever, colds, infections

- Drug abuse, especially with "uppers" such as PCP (phencyclidine hydrochloride) and amphetamines

- Drug withdrawal from "downers," barbiturates, Valium or alcohol

- Missed medication dosages

- Drug toxicity (too much medication)

- Sensory stimulation such as: sudden loud noise or sudden flashing lights

- Many more things too numerous to mention, and others that are still unknown

Appendix 2: Seizure Emergency Checklist

1. Do not restrain! This can make the seizure more severe.

2. Stay nearby.

3. Speak kindly.

4. If the person is moving around, remove dangerous, sharp or hot objects from the area.

5. Stand behind the person and gently guide him or her away from danger.

6. If the person shakes or falls, turn the head or whole body to the side so that saliva can drain from the mouth.

7. Force nothing between the teeth. The outdated practice of putting an object in the mouth to prevent the person from swallowing the tongue is not appropriate. The tongue cannot be swallowed. A hard object can increase the damage to the tongue from biting. A soft object can become lodged in the throat, causing suffocation.

8. If stiffness or shaking continue for over 10 minutes or if the person seems to pass from one seizure to another without regaining consciousness, call an ambulance.

9. Time and observe the person's actions before, during and after a seizure, for a medical report.

10. When the seizure is over, let the person rest and do not show alarm, as this only adds to his or her embarrassment and nervousness.

Appendix 3: Suggested Books for Further Reading

Factual Books on Epilepsy

Adult

Dictionary of Epilepsy, by Professor H. Gastut and others, World Health Organization Publications Centre, Geneva, Switzerland

Epilepsy, by Middleton, Attwell and Walsh, Little, Brown and Co., Boston-Toronto

Epilepsy, A Medical Handbook for Physicians, Nurses, Teachers, Parents, Nogan, Carmi Corp., fort Worth, Texas

The Epilepsy Fact Book, by Sands and Minters, Charles Scribner's Sons, NY

The Falling Sickness, by O. Temkin, John Hopkins University Press

Having Epilepsy, by Schneider and Conrad, Temple Univ. Press, Philadelphia, PA

Learning About Epilepsy, by William B. Svoboda, M.D., University Park Press, Baltimore

Rusty's Story, by Carol Gino, Bantam Books

Seizures, Epilepsy and Your Child, by J. C. Lagos, Harper & Row

The Spirit Catches You and You Fall Down, by Anne Fadiman, Farrar Straus & Giroux

Youth

Epilepsy, by A. Silverstein, Lippincott, CO

Novels About Epilepsy

Elementary

What Difference Does It Make, Danny?, by Helen Young, E. P. Dutton

What If They Knew?, by Patricia Hermes, Dell Publishing

Junior & Senior High School

A Handful of Stars, by Barbara Girion, Scribner's Sons

Adult

The Children's Ward, by Howard Weiner, M.D., Putnam's Sons

Books on Stress Management

Guide to Stress Management, by L. John Mason, Ph.D., Celestial Arts, Berkeley, CA

Mind As Healer, Mind As Slayer, by Kenneth R. Pelletier, Delacorte Press, NY

The Relaxation Response, by Herbert Benson, M.D., Avon, NY

Books on Yoga

Integral Yoga Hatha, by Yogiraz Sri Swami Satchidananda, Holt, Rinehart and Winston, NY, Chicago, San Francisco

Light On Yoga, by B.K.S. Iyengar, Schocken Books, NY

The Light of Yoga Beginner's Manual, by Alice Christensen and David Rankin, Simon and Schuster, NY

Books on Health and General Well-Being

A Symphony In The Brain, by Jim Robbins, Atlantic Monthly Press, ISBN 0-87113-807-7

Beyond Biofeedback, by Elmer and Alyce Green, Delacorte Press, Seymour

Lawrence, NY

Quantum Healing, by Deepak Chopra, M.D., Bantam New Age Books

Gifts From Eykis, by Wayne Dyer, Pocket Books, NY

High Level Wellness, by Donald B. Ardell, Bantam Books, NY

Inner Balance, The Power of Holistic Healing, ed. By Mark Bricklin, Rodale, Emmaus, Penn.

Books on Music and Healing

The Mozart Effect, Don Campbell, Avon Books, New York

Music, The Brain, and Ecstasy, Robert Jourdain, Avon Books, New York

The Healing Energies of Music, Hal A. Lingerman, Theological Publishing House, Wheaton, Ill.

The Healing Sound of Music, Kate & Richard Mucci, Findhorn Press, Tallahassee, Florida

Books on Drug Information

Physician's Desk Reference, Charles E. Baker, Jr., Publisher, Medical Economics Co., a Litton Division, Oradell, NJ

The Essential Guide to Prescription Drugs, by James W. Long, M.D., Harper and Row

Appendix 4: Finding Out More

Organizations For Epilepsy

Epilepsy Foundation of America: www.epilepsyfoundation.org

The International League Against Epilepsy: www.ilae-epilepsy.org

Searching the Internet

Go to your favorite search engine: type in "epilepsy".

Where to Find a Neurofeedback Practitioner

Ask for EEG Biofeedback (Neurofeedback) Practitioners in your area.

AAPB (Association for Applied Psychophysiological Biofeedback, 10200 W. 44TH Ave., Ste.304, Wheat Ridge, CO 80033-2840, www.aapb.org, e-mail: AAPB@resourcecenter.com. Phone: 1-800-477-8892

BCIA (Biofeedback Certification Institute of America), 10200 W. 44th Ave., Ste. 310, Wheat Ridge, CO 80033-2840, www.bcia.org, email: bcia@resourcecenter.com. Phone: (303)420-2902

Society for Neuronal Regulation, 394 Road 34, Marino, CO 80741, www.snr-jnt.org. Phone: 1-800-488-3867

Glossary

Many of these words have multiple meanings and uses. This glossary focuses on the definitions that relate to epilepsy and the topics covered in this book.

Absence Seizure: Petit Mal Seizure. A seizure characterized by momentary lapse of consciousness or inattention.

Acetylcholine: An ester of choline usually present in the body. It transmits an impulse from one nerve fiber to another.

Active Epilepsy: Seizures uncontrolled for a period of five years without medicine.

Acute: Coming on rapidly, with severe symptoms and a short course; opposite of chronic.

Adaptive Behavior: A subconscious means by which a person adjusts to his or her environment.

Adrenal: *See* epinephrine.

Adversive Seizure: A focal seizure in which the eyes, head, or trunk often turn to one side. One arm sometimes remains raised during the seizure.

Aerobic Exercise: Any activity which will raise the heartbeat, increasing oxygen in the body.

Affect: The feeling experienced with an emotion.

Affective Seizure: A seizure, usually focal or temporal lobe, accompanied by emotional reactions (crying, laughing, etc.).

Affirmation: A positive statement repeated to yourself, either silently or out loud.

Agnosia: An organic brain disorder which results in the inability to recognize and interpret sensory impressions.

Akinetic Seizure: A generalized seizure, usually in children, characterized by loss of muscle control. Often there is a sudden falling forward or loss of consciousness, of widely varying duration. Also known as Drop Epilepsy.

Allergen: Anything which causes an allergic reaction. Allergens may be foods, drugs, infectious agents, physical substances, contactants and inhalants.

Allergy: A changed body reaction to a certain substance (allergen) which in nonsensitive people will, in similar amounts, have no effect.

Alpha Rhythm: Fairly large, rhythmic brain waves of approximately 8 – 12 Hz, as recorded in an EEG; associated with relaxation.

Amino Acid: The building blocks of protein. The body breaks down complex proteins into amino acids, then uses the amino acids for growth or metabolism. There are 22 amino acids, eight of them classified as the essential amino acids, the other 14 classified as nonessential. The amino acids cannot be manufactured by the human body, and must be obtained from the diet.

Amnesia: Loss of memory, either partial or total. Functional inability to recall the past.

Amphetamines: A group of synthetic central nervous system stimulants which increase general activity, suppress appetite, and which may generate feelings of well-being. Used medically as anti-depressant and anti-obesity drugs.

Amplitude: The strength or intensity of the brain wave signals in regard to EEG biofeedback.

Analeptic: A substance that has a convulsive-producing or stimulatory agent.

Anoxia: A condition caused by a deficiency of oxygen in the blood, which leads to inadequate tissue functioning. Also known as hypoxia.

Anti-convulsant: A medicine, agent, diet or procedure used to control seizures.

Anxiety: A generalized feeling of apprehension or worry without apparent cause, related to fear.

Apathy: A feeling of listlessness or indifference, in which the person loses interest in him/herself. One of the consequences of frustration.

Aphasia: A loss of ability to name common objects or to pronounce words. It sometimes involves written expression.

Arteriogram: An X-ray of an artery after injecting an opaque substance for clarity. When used in the diagnosis of epilepsy, it is an X-ray of arteries in the brain.

Asana: A comfortable pose; a stretching posture in yoga.

Asymptomatic: Showing no symptoms.

Ataxia: Loss of muscular coordination, especially with voluntary muscular movements.

Atonic: Loss of muscle tone.

Atonic Seizure: A generalized seizure, usually brief, where there is a sagging of the head, body or limbs.

Atrophy: A reduction in size or wasting of a structure by disease, injury or disuse.

Attention: The process of focusing perception on a single event or object. Concentration.

Audiogenic Seizure: A convulsion induced by high-frequency sound waves.

Auditory: Pertaining to the sense of hearing.

Aura: The sensation or "feeling" which precedes a seizure. The sensations may be sensory, motor or autonomic. The aura is actually the seizure discharge beginning.

Autogenic Phrases: The phrases which you say to yourself to achieve a state of relaxation, such as, "I am very relaxed."

Automatism: Automatic behavior or actions without conscious purpose or knowledge. Complicated acts may be carried out without any recollection or awareness of the acts.

Autonomic Manifestations: Motor or sensory manifestations that often occur along with generalized seizures. They sometimes occur as an aura, and may involve perspiration, hypertension, vomiting, loss of bowel control, etc.

Autonomic Nervous System (ANS): The part of the nervous system involved with the control of involuntary functions. It controls the functioning of the glands, blood vessels, smooth muscles and the heart.

Awareness: Consciousness, alertness. A state of knowledge or understanding of internal events or environment.

Axon: The portion of a neuron that transmits impulses away from the cell to other neurons. *See* dendrite, neuron.

Barbiturate: Any drug, such as phenobarbitol, which acts as a central nervous system (CNS) depressant and sedative. Induces drowsiness and muscular relaxation.

Beta Rhythm: Brain waves of approximately 13 Hz or above, faster than alpha waves, as recorded in an EEG. Most often observed when the person is alert.

Bilateral: Pertaining to two sides. When referring to epilepsy, meaning both sides of the head.

Biofeedback: The feedback of biological information. A training procedure where information concerning the functioning of internal organs is obtained, usually through the use of electronic equipment. Because of the information, the trainee learns to control certain body functions, such as brain waves, skin temperature or muscle tension. *See* neurofeedback.

Birth Trauma: An injury which occurs during birth.

Brain Stem: The portion of the brain lying near the core of the brain. All of the brain except the cerebrum and the cerebellum.

Brain Wave: The rhythmical electrical activity or discharges of the brain. *See* electroencephalogram.

Bruxism: Grinding the teeth, especially during sleep.

Calcium: An essential mineral necessary for bone formation and development. Must be taken with magnesium. Deficiency leads to hyperexcitability of the neuromuscular system.

CATScan (Computerized Axial Tomograph): A testing method to detect tiny variations in tissue density which are not obvious with conventional X-ray techniques. Highly sensitive X-ray detectors along with advanced computer data processing produce a recording of information for future use.

Cataplexy: A condition where the person becomes immobile, loses muscle tone and falls to the floor. Caused by sudden emotional shock.

Central Fissure: A deep groove in the brain which begins in the middle of each cerebral hemisphere and runs downward.

It separates the frontal from the parietal lobe.

Central Nervous System (CNS): The brain and spinal cord.

Cerebellar Ataxia: The outermost layer of the brain. It contains motor, association and sensory areas.

Cerebellum: The portion of the brain in the lower region of the cranium that controls balance, motor coordination and muscle tone.

Cerebral Cortex: The outermost layer of the brain. It contains motor, association and sensory areas.

Cerebral Hemisphere: *See* cerebrum.

Cerebral Lesion: Any form of pathological abnormality of the brain.

Cerebrospinal Fluid: A lymphlike fluid within the spinal cord and ventricles of the brain.

Cerebrum: The largest part of the brain located in the upper region of the cranium. It consists of two hemispheres separated by a deep longitudinal fissure. The cerebrum is the seat of consciousness. It interprets sensory impulses and all voluntary muscular activities. It is the center of the higher mental faculties such as learning, memory, reasoning, intelligence, judgment and the emotions.

Chorea: A widespread twitching or jerking of muscles.

Chromosomes: The carriers of the genes within the nucleus of the cell.

Chronic: Long drawn out. When applied to a disorder, not acute, continual, recurring.

Cirrhosis: A chronic disease of the liver which can be caused by one of the following: poisons, drugs, nutritional deficiency or previous inflammation.

Clinical: Referring to the professional observation and treatment of patients.

Clinical Psychologist: A psychologist with a Ph.D. degree, trained in the diagnosis and treatment of emotional and behavioral problems, as well as mental disorders.

Clonic: Jerking movements of the extremities (arms and legs) or body.

CNS: *See* central nervous system.

Cognitive: Referring to mental processes such as judgment, thinking, comprehension, etc.

Communication: The transmission of energy, signals, information or messages.

Complex Partial Seizure: Also called Temporal Lobe or Psychomotor Seizure. International Classification of Epileptic Seizure meaning complex symptomatology (generally with impairment of consciousness). Usually accompanied by strange, subjective feelings such as illusions, visions, strangeness or familiarity, or involuntary movements.

Concussion: A general term meaning a loss of consciousness due to a blow on the head.

Congenital: Present at birth, but acquired during fetal development; not inherited.

Contraction: A shortening, tensing or tightening of a muscle.

Consultation: Diagnosis and suggested treatment by two or more physicians. A consulting physician or surgeon is one who is contacted for advice.

Convulsion: An involuntary series of muscle contractions and relaxations. Also known as a seizure, fit or spell.

Corpus Callosum: A large nerve tract connecting the right and left sides of the cerebrum, allowing coordination of the functions of each side or hemisphere.

Cortex: *See* cerebral cortex.

Cortical Seizure: A partial or focal seizure caused by excessive discharge in one part of the cerebral cortex. These seizures, though focal, sometimes spread and become generalized.

Cranial Nerves: The twelve motor and sensory nerves that connect directly with the brain.

Cryptogenic Epilepsy: *See* idiopathic epilepsy.

Déjà vu: The illusion of familiarity in a strange place. The impression that a new situation has been previously seen or experienced.

Delta Waves: Very slow brain waves of approximately .05 – 3 Hz when recorded with EEG biofeedback. Produced in deep, dreamless sleep.

Dendrite: The fiber of a neuron which receives impulses from other neurons. *See also* Axon, Neuron.

Depression: A state of despondency, melancholy or dejection, feeling "blue," "down." Feelings of hopelessness, inadequacy and pessimism about the future.

Diagnosis: The procedure by which the nature of a disease or condition is determined.

Diaphragm: A thin membrane wall separating the abdomen from the cavity of the chest.

Disorientation: Inability to be aware of time or people, or to estimate location or direction.

Diurnal Seizure: A daytime seizure when the person is awake, in contrast to a nocturnal seizure when the person is asleep.

Dopamine: A neurotransmitter of the central nervous system. It is synthesized from an amino acid, then converted into norepinephrine. *See also* neurotransmitter, norepinephrine.

Drop Epilepsy: *See* akinetic seizure.

Dysarthria: Impairment of speech because of organic disorders in the nervous system.

Dysgraphia: Writing difficulties as a result of a neurological disorder.

EEG: *See* electroencephalogram.

Electrode: A conductor through which energy enters or leaves a medium, such as with an EEG.

Electroencephalogram (EEG): The diagram, print-out or findings from an EEG (brain wave activity).

Encephalitis: Inflammation of the brain, often as a result of infection. Symptoms may include severe headache, fever, stiffness of the neck, and peculiar symptoms such as euphoria, sleepiness or giddiness.

Encephalon: The brain.

Encephalopathy: Any disease of the brain.

Encopresis: Involuntary discharge of the stool.

Enuresis: Involuntary discharge of urine.

Enuretic Seizure: Enuresis associated with seizure. Not the same as simple nocturnal enuresis (bedwetting).

Epilepsy: A disorder characterized by recurring attacks of central nervous system dysfunction, with or without lack of consciousness.

Epileptic Coma: An unconscious state which follows generalized seizures or status epilepticus.

Epileptic Confusion: A confused state which occurs during or following seizures.

Epileptic Discharge: An abnormal electrical discharge from cerebral neurons in some people with epilepsy.

Epileptic Fugue: Gestural or ambulatory movements of an automatic nature, frequently following a generalized seizure, and often lasting for up to an hour. Characterized by amnesia and flight.

Epileptic Hallucinations: Various perceptions of smell, taste, feeling, etc., that follow an attack. Similar to the aura at the beginning of a seizure.

Epileptogenic: A condition in a person which induces seizure activity, for example, brain lesions.

Epileptologist: A neurologist who specializes in the treatment of epilepsy.

Epinephrine: A substance produced by the adrenal medulla which enables the body to cope with emergency situations. There is increased heart rate and blood pressure, a transfer of blood from the skin and stomach to the skeletal muscles, and digestion is inhibited. In effect, it prepares the person for fight or flight emergency action. Also known as adrenaline.

Etiology: The cause of a disorder, condition or disease.

Euphoria: A state of well-being or elation. Common among toxic states and organic brain disease.

Excitable: Pertaining to highly reactive nervous tissue. Large, peripheral neurons are highly excitable.

Excitatory Synapse: A synapse at which the neurotransmitter changes the membrane permeability of the receiving cell in the direction of depolarization.

Extremity: The terminal or ending part of anything. An arm or leg.

Extroversion: Interest in other people and the environment. Often referred to as "outgoingness." The opposite of introversion or shyness.

Familial: In regard to or characteristic of a certain family, thought to be inherited.

Fatigue: A feeling of exhaustion, weariness or tiredness.

Febrile: Relating to or having a fever.

Febrile Convulsion: An attack brought about by a fever. Occurs mostly between the ages of six months and five years.

Fit: *See* seizure.

Focal Motor Seizure: Classical Jacksonian form of epilepsy, in which there is no loss of consciousness. Starts in one part of the motor area of the cortex and spreads to involve the rest of the motor strip. Caused by abnormal electrical discharge in one part of the brain, affecting the part of the body controlled by that part of the brain.

Focal Sensory Seizure: Involves a certain part of the brain where sensations of various types are appreciated, such as visual, somatic, auditory, olfactory, vertiginous or abdominal.

Folate: A salt of folic acid.

Folic Acid: A member of the B vitamin complex. Essential for normal blood formation, and is involved in many important metabolic processes. Good sources are spinach, asparagus, liver, wheat bran, broccoli. Extremely large amounts of folic acid may cause anti-convulsant drugs to lose their effectiveness.

Food Supplement: Any substance designed to supply nutrients that may be lacking in the diet.

Free-Floating Anxiety: Fear, apprehension or anxiety not attached to specific objects or situations. The person often cannot explain this continuing condition.

Frequency: In regard to neurofeedback (EEG biofeedback), the speed of the brain wave signals.

Frontal Lobe: The area of the central cortex serving as the brain's center for complex associations.

Gamma-Aminobutryic Acid (GABA): A substance that changes the normal balance of the nerve cells.

Gastritis: Inflammation of the stomach characterized by nausea, pain or tenderness, and vomiting.

Gastrointestinal: Pertaining to the intestine and stomach.

Gene, Dominant: A gene that produces an effect in the offspring, even if it is not matched by a like gene in the mate's chromosome.

Gene, Multiple: A gene whose individual effects are small. It combines with others to produce additive effects.

Gene, Recessive: A gene that produces its effect only if it is matched by a like gene of the other chromosome of the mate.

Generalized Seizures: Seizures that result from a generalized, nonfocal, electrical discharge in the brain (not just a specific part of the brain). The two most common forms are absence (petit mal) and tonic-clonic (grand mal). *The International Classification of Epileptic Seizures* lists the following types of seizures:

* Absence (petit mal)

* Bilateral massive epileptic myoclonus

* Infantile Spasms

* Clonic Seizures (the jerking part of a seizure)

* Tonic Seizures (the stiffening part of a seizure)

* Tonic-clonic Seizures (grand mal)

* Atonic Seizures

* Akinetic Seizures

Gestation: The period of pregnancy.

Gingival Hyperplasia: Swelling of the gums, often caused by certain anti-convulsants.

Glia: The connective tissue elements in the brain.

Glucose: The most important carbohydrate in body metabolism. Formed during digestion and absorbed from the intestine into the blood. When it passes through the liver, excess glucose is changed into glycogen and stored for future use.

Glutamic Acid: One of the nonessential amino acids found in protein foods. It can be used as a fuel by brain cells.

Glutamine: *See* Glutamic Acid.

Glycogen: The form in which carbohydrate is stored in the body until it is converted into sugar when needed by the tissues. It assists in performing muscular work or generating body heat.

Grand Mal Seizure: Generalized tonic-clonic seizure. A major seizure consisting of alternate stiffening (tonic) and jerking (clonic). There is loss of consciousness.

Gray Matter: The neural substance of the brain and spinal cord, made up mostly of cell bodies.

Gustatory: Pertaining to the sense of taste.

Hallucination: False perception unrelated to reality. Similar to déjà vu or visualization. May be visual, auditory, olfactory, etc. Formed hallucinations are a type of complex partial seizures.

Hemiparesis: Weakness of muscles on one side of the body.

Hemiplegia: Paralysis of one side of the body.

Hemispherectomy: An operation removing a cerebral hemisphere.

Hereditary: Transmitted from parent to offspring through the genes. This transmission of genetic characteristics is a function of the chromosomes and genes.

Hertz (Hz): The wave frequency measuring sound waves, EEG brain waves, etc. Measured in cycles per second.

Homeopathy: A system of medicine in which disease is treated with extremely small quantities of substances which would themselves produce the symptoms of the disease in normal dosages. Modern homeopathy was founded by Hahemann over 170 years ago.

Hormone: A substance formed by an organ or by certain cells of an organ which circulates in the body and produces a specific effect in some other part of the body.

Hydrocephalus: An accumulation of cerebrospinal fluid in the cranium. This can cause an enlargement of the head in infancy. If not arrested early, it will result in mental retardation.

Hyperactivity: Excessive, uncontrollable activity.

Hypertension: High blood pressure. The most common symptoms include fatigue, nervousness, dizziness, headaches, insomnia, and rapid heart-beat.

Hyperventilation: Excessively fast or deep breathing resulting in an excess of oxygen in the blood. Sometimes causes buzzing in the head, tingling, momentary blackouts or convulsions.

Hypnosis: The responsive state achieved following a typical hypnotic induction or its equivalent.

Hypnotic Induction: The procedure used in establishing hypnosis in a responsive person. It frequently involves relaxation and stimulated imagination.

Hypoglycemia: Low blood sugar. A condition often caused by an excess of sugar and other carbohydrates in the diet, or by a tumor on the pancreas. After eating food rich in carbohydrates, the blood sugar level often tends to rise rapidly and drops quickly, resulting in hypoglycemia.

Hypothalamus: A portion of the brain that controls, activates and integrates autonomic mechanisms and endocrine activity. It regulates body temperature, sleep, water balance and food intake.

Hypsarrhythmia: A common EEG pattern seen in children with myoclonic epilepsy.

Hysterical Seizure: An attack resembling a seizure but with no abnormal discharge in the brain. It is often psychological in origin. Most hysterical seizures occur in people who also have regular seizures.

Hz: *See* Hertz.

Ictal: Pertaining to a seizure.

Idiopathic: Pertaining to conditions which cannot be clearly explained, or disease without recognizable cause.

Idiopathic Epilepsy: A term applied to recurring seizures when there is no known organic cause and the EEG is normal.

Incontinence: Loss of sphincter control, with the result being inability to retain feces or urine.

Infantile Epilepsy: Seizures in newborns and infants. Believed to be caused by such things as incomplete cerebral maturation, or a predisposition. Seizures are of several types.

Infantile Myoclonic Seizures: Massive seizures in babies, consisting of spasms, unconsciousness, and autonomic movements. Believed to be caused by brain malfunction of unknown origin.

Infant Spasms: A seizure disorder which occurs during the first year of life. Characterized by tonic seizures.

Insulin: A hormone secreted by the pancreas. It is necessary for the proper metabolism of glucose (blood sugar) and to maintain the proper blood sugar level.

Interbrain: The diencephalons, consisting of the thalamus, epithalamus and hypothalamus.

Interictal: Pertaining to activity between seizures.

Introversion: Reduced interest in other people and the environment. Preoccupation with self. Opposite of extroversion.

Involuntary Movement: A movement which is made in spite of an effort not to make it.

Jacksonian Seizure: *See* focal motor seizure.

Jamais vu: The illusion of hearing music, perceiving tastes or smells or recalling vivid scenes.

Lecithin: A mixture of phospholipids found in all plants and animals. In humans lecithin plays an important part in a healthy nervous system.

Left Hemisphere: The left cerebral hemisphere. Controls the right side of the body, and for most people, speech and other logical, cognitive activities.

Lesion: A change in tissue as a result of injury or disease.

Libido: The energy of the sexual or erotic instinct.

Lobe: A fairly well defined section of an organ. Principal lobes of the cerebrum are frontal, parietal, occipital and temporal lobes.

Lobectomy: Removal of a lobe of the brain (cerebrum).

Lobotomy: Brain surgery in which certain brain nerve fibers are cut to reduce tension and stress for psychiatric patients. Used in the past for severe epilepsy patients.

Localized Functions: Behavior controlled by certain areas of the brain. For instance, vision is localized in the occipital lobes toward the back of the head.

Log: A record of performance.

Long-Term Memory (LTM): Permanent memory or memory which endures for long periods of time, possibly for life, as opposed to short-term memory.

Low Blood Sugar: *See* hypoglycemia.

Low Seizure Threshold: Having a low tolerance, and thus a high susceptibility to seizures.

Lysine: One of the eight essential amino acids.

Magnesium: An essential mineral widely distributed throughout the body. It is essential for proper calcium and vitamin C metabolism. It must be taken with calcium. Good sources are cereals and sesame seeds.

Manganese: A mineral necessary for the nerve transmitter system, tissue respiration, reproduction, and proper glandular function, especially milk formation in nursing women. It is found in green leafy vegetables, whole grains, beans, peas, nuts, eggs and red meats.

Medulla: The lower portion of the brain above the spinal cord, in front of the cerebellum. It is an aid for regulating heartbeat, blood pressure and breathing.

Meditation: A sustained effort at contemplative thinking or concentration. The goal being either deeper thinking or detached non-thinking.

Megavitamin Therapy: Vitamins which are given in massive doses.

Memory: The function involved in reliving past experiences. The totality of a specific past experience. The memory process is measured by recall, reproduction and relearning.

Meningitis: Inflammation or swelling of the membranes of the brain or spinal cord. Thought to be a frequent cause of epilepsy. Also called Encephalitis.

Menarche: The first menstrual period for a girl. *See* menstruation.

Menstruation: The cyclic, approximately monthly, discharge of blood and material from the uterus in mature females.

Mephenytoin (Mesantoin): A second-line drug, similar to phenytoin, used in the treatment of focal-onset and tonic-clonic seizures.

Mephobarbital (Mebaral): A barbiturate sometimes used as an anti-convulsant.

Metabolism: The chemical changes which go on in the living organism, providing energy for functions and the building of tissues.

Methsuximide (Celontin): A second-line drug structurally related to ethosuximide. Commonly used for absence seizures, myoclonic jerks and atonic seizures.

Mono-Drug Therapy: Treatment of a disorder, specifically, epilepsy, with a single anti-convulsant drug.

Motor: Referring to muscular movement, either conscious or unconscious.

Motor Area: An area in the brain lying in front of the central fissure. Stimulation often results in motor, or movement, responses.

Multiple Sclerosis: A progressive and degenerative disease of the central nervous system. It is brought on by a hardening of the tissues of the spinal cord and/or brain.

Musicogenic Epilepsy: An unusual type of partial, temporal lobe seizure brought on by one's emotional reaction to certain types of music.

Myelitis: Inflammation of the spinal cord.

Myoclonic Seizure: A generalized convulsive seizure, usually of short duration, characterized by muscular spasms of the whole body.

Mysoline: *See* Primidone.

Myth: A traditional, false belief which is widely accepted among the population.

Narcolepsy: A disorder characterized by extreme sleepiness during the day (cataplexy). It is occasionally accompanied by hallucinations just before or after sleep.

Nerve Impulse: An electrochemical excitation which passes along nerve cells.

Nervous System: The totality of neural tissues.

Nervousness: A state of restlessness with heightened emotionality. There are often signs of muscular tremor, tenseness and overactivity.

Neural Discharge: The excitation and propagation of a localized disturbance in a neuron or nervous center.

Neural Excitation: The process whereby a state of irritability is initiated in a neuron by an outside stimulus.

Neurologist: A medical doctor (physician) who specializes in the diagnosis and treatment of disorders of the nervous system.

Neurology: The science and study of the nervous system and brain.

Neuromuscular: Pertaining to the relationship between nerves and muscles.

Neuron: The single cell which is the elementary building block of the nervous system, with the function of transmitting impulses. Also called nerve cell.

Neuronal Discharge: The discharge of one or more nerve impulses.

Neuropsychiatrist: One who combines the practice of neurology and psychiatry. A physician who specializes in psychiatric or nervous disorders related to the nervous system.

Neurosurgeon: A physician who specializes in brain surgery.

Neurotransmitter: A chemical that transmits signals between the nerve cells and the brain.

Nocturnal Seizures: Seizures which occur during sleep.

Norepinephrine (Noradrenalin): A substance produced by the adrenal medulla which enables the body to cope with emergency situations. Its effects are similar to epinephrine. The only difference is that norepinephrine constricts the blood vessels, whereas epinephrine constricts some and dilates others.

Nutrition: All of the processes involved with normal growth and development. Nourishment.

Nystagmus: An involuntary, jerking movement of the eyes.

Occipital Lobe: The area of the cerebral cortex located at the back of the brain. It is the primary center for vision.

Ocular: Pertaining to the eye.

Olfactory: Pertaining to the sense of smell.

Organic: Pertaining to the structure of organs in contrast to their function.

Organic Involvement: Any structural condition which affects mental, motor, or communicative functions, caused by injury to an organ such as the brain. For example, epilepsy.

Overprotection: The tendency on the part of parents or others to shelter an individual excessively, providing protection from physical and psychological harm to such a degree that the individual fails to become independent.

Palsy: Impairment of motor function as a result of brain injury.

Paraplegia: Paralysis of the lower half of the body.

Paresis: Slight or partial motor paralysis.

Parietal Lobe: The division of the cerebral hemisphere behind the central sulcus and in front of the occipital lobe. The parietal lobe contains somesthetic centers.

Paroxysmal: Referring to a sudden, periodic attack or recurrence of symptoms.

Partial Seizure: A focal, localized seizure, often involving only one side of the body.

Partial Complex Seizure: *See* complex partial seizure.

Passive Volition: Performing or accomplishing a task with very little active direction. "Letting it happen."

Pediatrician: A physician who specializes in the care of children.

Pediatric Neurologist: A neurologist specializing in the care of children with disorders of the nervous system.

Perception: The process of selecting, organizing and integrating sensory data.

Perseverance: A tendency to continue an ongoing behavior in spite of opposition.

Petit Mal Seizure: *See* absence seizure.

Phenobarbital: The oldest anti-convulsant.

Phenothiazine: The basic neuromuscular transmitter to activate the muscles. An important chemical in the transmission of impulses from one nerve fiber to another across a synaptic junction.

Phenylalanine: An amino acid which is a neurotransmitter to activate the muscles. An important chemical in the transmission of impulses from one nerve fiber to another across a synaptic junction.

Phenytoin (Dilantin): An anti-convulsant drug for focal-onset secondarily generalized tonic-clonic and generalized-onset seizures.

Phobia: A strong, persistent and irrational fear, sometimes accompanied by compulsive avoidance mechanisms.

Photophobia: Fear of or intolerance to light.

Physician: A doctor of medicine.

Pituitary Gland: An endocrine gland attached to the base of the brain. The hormones it secretes regulate growth, reproduction and various metabolic activities. It is the master gland of the body.

Placebo: A preparation, often in pill form, which has no organic or proven benefit as a medicine. There are often beneficial results because the patient thinks the placebo has value.

Plaque: A gummy mass of microorganisms which grows around the teeth. Regular self-care of the teeth will help to prevent it. Some anti-convulsant medications increase this growth.

Pneumoencephalogram: An X-ray of the head after air or gas has been substituted for spinal fluid. It is helpful for outlining the brain by radiography.

Postictal: Following a seizure.

Post-Traumatic Epilepsy: Epilepsy following a severe injury to the head.

Preictal: Preceding a seizure.

Preventive Medicine: A branch of medicine that focuses on the prevention of disease and the maintenance of good health. All systems of medicine incorporate preventive medicine to some degree.

Primidone (Mysoline): An anti-convulsant drug used for generalized tonic-clonic and focal-onset seizures.

Prognosis: Prediction based upon current evidence.

Progressive Relaxation: A method for achieving total relaxation by tensing, then relaxing, various parts of the body, part by part.

Prophylaxis: Any preventive treatment of a disorder.

Protein: Any of a group of complex nitrogenous compounds that can be broken down into amino acids. Proteins are found in all living organisms. As a food, protein is an absolutely essential nutrient, especially for people with epilepsy.

Psychiatrist: A medical doctor specializing in the treatment and prevention of mental disorders.

Psychic Seizure: A focal (partial) seizure identified with certain emotional stimulation.

Psychologist: An individual trained in the diagnosis and treatment of emotional and behavioral problems as well as mental disorders.

Psychomotor Seizure: *See* complex partial seizure.

Psychosis: A severe emotional disorder, resulting in loss of contact with reality.

Psychosomatic: Pertaining to the relation of mind and body. Pertaining to processes that are both somatic (bodily) and psychic (mental) in nature.

Psychotherapy: Individual or group treatment of various psychological problems by a therapist.

Pyridoxine: *See* vitamin B6.

Reading Epilepsy: A form of seizure believed induced by the rapid eye movements needed in reading, or by the intellectual or emotional reaction to the stimulation while reading.

Recommended Daily Allowance (RDA): The recommended amount of a nutrient to be taken daily by a normal, healthy human being. The RDA for each essential nutrient was established by the United States Food and Drug Administration (FDA).

Reflex Epilepsy: Seizures brought on by sensory stimulation, such as visual, auditory, smell, etc.

Reflex Inhibition: Pertaining to the prevention or inhibition of a seizure because of sensory stimulation. The opposite of reflex epilepsy.

Rehabilitation: The restoration to normal, or to as satisfactory a status as possible, of a person who has been injured or who has experienced severe problems.

Relaxation: A state of low tension without strong emotions. The return of a muscle to a resting state following contraction.

Remission: A time when the symptoms are not present.

Secondary Epilepsy: Seizures which have been acquired, i.e. toxic or metabolic.

Seizure: A sudden attack of abnormal electrical discharge in the brain causing a disturbance in the functioning of the brain for a short time and affecting body systems.

Seizure Focus: The particular place in the brain where there is abnormal electrical discharge.

Self-Actualization: The ideal state, in which an individual accepts oneself as functioning at capacity.

Self-Concept: An individual's total opinion of him or herself.

Self-Esteem: To appreciate and value one's self. Self-confidence.

Self-Induced Seizure: A generalized seizure, brought on deliberately often by photic stimulation or hyperventilation. More often found in children than adults.

Sensorimotor Rhythm (SMR): 12 – 15 Hz brain wave rhythm. Biofeedback (neurofeedback) training for SMR often leads to decreased seizure activity for individuals.

Sensory Seizure: A partial (focal) seizure which is accompanied by sensations such as hallucinations.

Serotonin: A neurotransmitter found in the midbrain. It is believed to play a part in mental illness, especially in depression.

Short-Term Memory (STM): Memory that has short duration (usually a few seconds) and is of limited capacity. *See* also long-term memory.

Sodium Valproate: *See* valproic acid.

Solar Plexus: The network of nerves behind the stomach in the abdomen, in front of the diaphragm.

Somatic Nervous System: A division of the peripheral nervous system. It is made up of nerves that connect the brain and spinal cord with the sense receptors, muscles and body surface.

Spasm: A lengthy muscular contraction, sometimes used to describe a childhood seizure.

Spike: A term used in electroencephalography (EEG) to denote a triangular-shaped wave that is sudden in appearance. It is out of keeping with the background brain wave activity.

Spike-and-Slow-Wave Discharge: A burst of high-amplitude brain wave activity (EEG) of spikes and slow inhibitory waves. It is useful for diagnosing and spotting a seizure focus, and appears in between seizures.

Spinal Cord: The neural structure in the backbone that acts as a pathway for impulses to and from the brain.

Spinal Nerves: The 31 pairs of nerves which are attached to the spinal cord.

SSI (Supplemental Security Income): A government program providing cash benefits for needy people.

Status Epilepticus: A series of recurring seizures, with little or no time between seizures. Requires immediate medical attention; otherwise death can result. Often caused by too rapid a change in medication.

Stimulants: Psychoactive drugs that increase arousal. Amphetamines, cocaine and caffeine are examples.

Stimulus: Any energy capable of attracting, exciting or stimulating the nervous system.

Stress: Reactions of the body or mind to influences or stimuli (stressors) that tend to upset the normal balance. A sense of strain or emotional tension. External stressors may be positive or negative (pleasure, challenge, work responsibilities, change). Long-term, subtle stress can lead to illness.

Subclinical Epilepsy: Seizures so mild that they often go unnoticed. They can usually be detected by irregular EEG (brain wave) activity or by perceptual psychometric testing.

Subcortical Epilepsy: Epilepsy that is thought to be caused by neural discharge in the subcortical parts of the brain.

Support: To provide encouragement, advice and concern for another individual.

Symptomatic Epilepsy: Epilepsy in which the seizures represent a symptom of a known, organic problem.

Synapse: The junction between two neurons.

Syndrome: A collection of symptoms which seem to be related.

Taurine: An amino acid, which acts as an inhibitory transmitter in the brain. It is important in the development and function of the brain.

Tegretol (Carbamazepine): An anti-convulsant for control of complex partial and secondarily generalized tonic-clonic seizures.

Temporal Lobe: A portion of the cerebral hemisphere in front of the occipital lobe, at the sides of the head. It is important for speech, hearing, perceptions and other associations.

Temporal Lobe Epilepsy: Focal or complex partial seizures, with the focus in or near the temporal lobe. They are usually preceded by an aura.

Thalamus: A mass of gray matter located just above the brain stem near the base of the cerebrum. It consists of two groups of nerve cell nuclei, one area acting as a sensory relay station, the other playing a role in sleep and waking.

Therapist: An individual who is trained in the treatment of disorders.

Therapy: Remedy or treatment.

Tofu: Soybean curd or soy cheese. A white food substance made by curdling soy milk with an acid. Tofu is rich in protein (important for those with epilepsy), and is often used as a meat substitute.

Transducer: A device, such as an electrode, which converts physiological (bodily) information into other forms of energy that can be recorded and measured. An electrode is a transducer in EEG biofeedback (neurofeedback).

Transmission: The sequential firing of one neuron in response to the firing of another.

Trauma: A severe emotional shock or problem, or a physical injury.

Tremor: An involuntary muscular movement or shaking of the body, often involving the limbs or head.

Tryptophan: An essential amino acid, which acts as an inhibitory neurotransmitter in the brain.

Tumor: An abnormal tissue growth or swelling.

Uncinate Seizure: A form of temporal lobe focal seizure. It is usually associated with smelling symptoms and/or hallucinations.

Unconscious: Pertaining to the state of a person who is not aware of the environment, such as from a faint or coma. Also, pertaining to all psychological or psychic processes which cannot be brought to awareness by ordinary means.

Unilateral Seizure: A focal seizure which involves only one side of the body.

United States Food and Drug Administration (FDA): A division of the United States Department of Health, Education and Welfare. It regulates many aspects of the food, drug and cosmetic industries. One of its main concerns is the safety and efficacy of drugs.

Valproic Acid (Depakene): An anti-convulsant used mainly for petit-mal (absence) seizures.

Ventricles: The communicating cavities in the brain that are continuous with the central canal of the spinal cord.

Vitamin: Any of a group of substances present in various foods in very small amounts, and required for normal growth and health. Even though they are not actual sources of energy, they are intricately involved with the processes of metabolism and respiration.

Vitamin B-3: *See* niacin or niacinamide.

Vitamin B-6: Pyridoxine. A water-soluble vitamin essential for amino acid and fatty acid metabolism. The other B vitamins, especially vitamin B-2 and magnesium, are required for the proper absorption of B-6.

Vitamin D: A fat-soluble vitamin essential for the utilization of calcium and phosphorus and for bone formation. Vitamin D is supplied by milk, fish liver oils and egg yolk. It can be manufactured in the body of exposure to sunlight is adequate.

White Matter: The substance found in the brain and spinal cord. It is composed of bundles of nerve fibers.

Yoga: Meaning "to yoke" or unity of being. In the Western world, the practice of physical postures, regulation of breathing, relaxation and meditation. Yoga in the spiritual sense is a system of beliefs and practices, the goal being to attain a union of the individual self with the Universal Being or Supreme Reality.

Zarontin: *See* ethosuximide.

Index

Index

P

Parietal lobe 14, 102, 113

Petit mal 17, 21, 31, 75–78, 107

Phenobarbitol 55, 101

Phenylalanine 58, 114

Positive statements 51

Primrose oil 58

Progressive relaxation 40, 52, 89

Pryridoxine 56

Psychomotor Seizure 8, 20, 21, 103, 115

R

Relaxation 30, 33, 34, 36, 40–42, 46, 48, 49, 51, 52, 67–69, 89, 100, 101, 108, 114, 119

S

Secondarily generalized seizure 20, 23

Seizure threshold 15, 17, 32, 39, 54, 55, 57, 58, 73, 90, 93, 110

Self-awareness 12

Self-esteem 7, 12, 81–88, 116

Sensorimotor rhythm 30, 32, 116

Simple partial seizure 18–20, 23

Sleep 9, 16, 22, 30, 31, 33, 39, 42, 52, 58, 67, 70, 78, 83, 90, 93, 102, 104, 109, 112, 118

Spike and wave pattern 8

Status epilepticus 23, 74, 105

Stress 7, 9, 12, 15, 16, 34, 39–52, 60, 62, 89, 90, 93, 110, 117

Stress management 7, 9, 41, 52, 123

Sugar 9, 16, 17, 53–55, 57, 90, 93, 107–109

Support groups 81

T

Taurine 59, 60, 117

Tegretol 74, 78, 117

Temporal lobe 8, 14, 17, 20, 31, 78, 99, 110, 111, 117, 118

Theta 30, 67, 122

Theta brain waves 30, 61, 122

Todd's phenomena 21

Tonic clonic seizure 22, 23, 78

Transmitter 57, 59, 110, 114, 117

Trauma 17, 29, 30, 39, 102, 118

Tryptophan 58, 59, 118

U

Unilateral seizure 18, 22, 118

V

Valium 16, 23, 66, 93

Vitamin B-1 58

Vitamin B-12 56, 58

Vitamin B-6 56, 58, 119

Vitamin C 57, 110

Vitamin D 57, 58, 61, 119

Y

Yoga 7, 9, 10, 40, 42–46, 48, 52, 61, 62, 89, 100

Z

Zarontin 78, 119

Inf<del>DATE DUE</del> Form

If you'd like a copy of this book for a friend, see your local bookstore, your favorite online bookseller, or order directly from Aura Publishing, either with this form, or online at www.epilepsyhealth.com.

Speaking/Performance Information:

❑   Please send me information about having Sally Fletcher speak to and/or give a healing concert for your organization, school, church or association.

Product Information:

Quant.	Title	List Price	Extended Price
	The Challenge of Epilepsy (book)	$17.95	$_____._____
	Healing from the Harp (CD)	$14.99	$_____._____
	Angels Awakening (CD)	$14.99	$_____._____
	Wedding Magic (CD)	$14.99	$_____._____
	A Christmas Miracle (CD)	$14.99	$_____._____
	Subtotal		$_____._____
	Sales Tax (California Residents, please add 7.5%)		$_____._____
	Shipping: $3.75 for the first book or CD, and $1.50 for each additional book or CD. These rates are for shipment to the US only. For destinations outside the US (including Canada), please call or email for shipping information.		$_____._____
	Total		$_____._____

Payment Information:

❑   My check or money order for $_____ is enclosed.

❑   Please charge my Visa or MasterCard

Visa or MasterCard # _____

Exp. Date _____

Signature: _____

Ship To:

Name: _____

Address: _____

City/State/Zip: _____

Phone: _____

E-mail: _____

Aura Publishing Company
P.O. Box 6776, San Rafael, CA 94903-6776
(415) 492-8034
www.epilepsyhealth.com   •   www.heavenlyharpist.com

About the Author

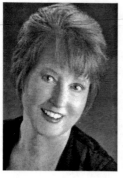

Sally Fletcher knows from experience what it is like to be diagnosed with a supposedly incurable disorder. For many years she had epileptic seizures—the result of a concussion from an ice skating fall. She couldn't undo the skating accident, and since medication didn't work for her, she found other solutions.

Her book, *The Challenge of Epilepsy,* describes the various methods that helped her take control of her life and end her seizures. She has been seizure-free with no medication for 18 years.

Sally's personal and professional experience with epilepsy has given her many answers for controlling seizures. For ten years she practiced as a certified biofeedback therapist, specializing in epilepsy, stress management, ADD (Attention Deficit Disorder) and ADHD (Attention Deficit Hyperactivity Disorder).

Recently, she has returned to her first love—music. She now performs and records music from the harp, sometimes adding her voice. Most of the music she plays at events is now from memory, which was definitely not possible before. The ethereal sound waves of her harp music provide relaxing, healing vibrations for the body, mind and soul.

In addition to concerts and other purely musical performances, Sally is a motivational speaker, inspiring people to face and overcome seemingly insurmountable obstacles. She weaves her harp playing through her talks to add entertainment, healing, relaxation and a "special" personal touch.

Her next book project, currently in progress, is *The Healing Power of Music.*